HEALTH TECHNOLOGY TRANSFER:
WHOSE RESPONSIBILITY?

XXIIIrd CIOMS Round Table Conference
Geneva, Switzerland
2-3 November 1989

Organized jointly with the World Health Organization

Edited by Z. Bankowski and G. L. Ada

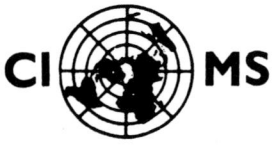

Geneva, 1990

CONFERENCE PROGRAMME COMMITTEE

Ada G. L. Professor, The John Curtin School of Medical Research, Canberra, Australia

Bankowski, Z. Council for International Organizations of Medical Sciences, Geneva, Switzerland

Fattorusso, V. Division of Drug Management and Policies, World Health Organization, Geneva, Switzerland

Hanson, G. Radiation Medicine, World Health Organization, Geneva, Switzerland

Mansourian, B. Office of Research Promotion and Development, World Health Organization, Geneva, Switzerland

Szczerban, J. Office of Research Promotion and Development, World Health Organization, Geneva, Switzerland

Vilardell, F. President, Council for International Organizations of Medical Sciences, Barcelona, Spain

TABLE OF CONTENTS

ACKNOWLEDGEMENTS

The Council for International Organizations of Medical Sciences is greatly indebted for their contribution in the preparation and organization of the Conference to Drs J. Szczerban and B. G. Mansourian of the Office of Research Promotion and Development of the World Health Organization and Drs V. Fattorusso, G. P. Hanson, V. M. Volodin and A. E. Wasunna of the then Division of Diagnostic, Therapeutic and Rehabilitative Technology of the World Health Organization.

Our special thanks are due to Professor G. L. Ada for his leadership and the efficient way in which he conducted the meeting, as well as for the preparation of the highlights of the Conference.

We thank very much Dr J. Gallagher for his assistance in the editing and preparation of this volume and Mrs Kathryn Chalaby-Amsler and Mrs C. Dübendorfer for their efficient work in the preparation of the Conference and of this volume.

v

INTRODUCTION

The conferences of the Council for International Organizations of Medical Sciences (CIOMS) are aimed at creating international and interdisciplinary forums to enable the scientific and lay communities to exchange views on topics of immediate concern, unhampered by administrative, political or other considerations. They discuss not only the scientific and technical basis of new developments in biology and medicine and other related areas, but also their social, economic, ethical, administrative and legal implications. Participants in these conferences are prominent representatives of different fields of medicine, the natural and the social sciences, philosophy, theology and law. This multidisciplinary approach is felt to be the best means of obtaining a comprehensive picture of issues that do not fall within the exclusive domain of any one profession.

One field of much topical concern in this respect is the transfer of high technology in health care from the highly industrialized countries to the less industrialized. The great variation among countries in social, economic, political and cultural characteristics raises serious ethical and human-value issues.

Health technology transfer, in its many forms, is a substantial component of many programmes of the World Health Organization (WHO) and has been the subject of a study by a subcommittee of the WHO Global Advisory Committee of Health Research.

In July 1985 the WHO Bi-Regional Conference on Technology Transfer in the Health Field, held in Tokyo, highlighted this problem. It referred to the special efforts of WHO in developing and improving health technology and in promoting and facilitating its transfer between countries. It called for a new type of partnership for health development, closely associated with socioeconomic development. The increasing interdependence of countries encompassed cooperation in solving health problems, particularly through the wise use of technology.

Advances in the basic medical sciences and their application to clinical medicine have opened up the way to new therapies and numerous specialties, demanding new and increasingly specific technologies. Medical research directed at the cure or alleviation of chronic diseases is resulting in new diagnostic, therapeutic and rehabilitative methods, and these will fundamentally influence health care in all countries, rich and poor. These methods have numerous present and future applications. Monoclonal antibodies, for example, will permit prompt and easy diagnosis of communicable and other diseases in developing countries and provide a valuable tool for epidemiological studies. DNA probes may permit the detection of pathogenic micro-organisms and the differentiation of active and latent infections. DNA recombinant technology has immense potential for the large-scale and economic production of vaccines.

Developments in diagnostic imaging technology—diagnostic ultrasound, computerized tomography, magnetic resonance imaging, and other techniques—are changing the face of diagnostic medicine.

Advances in materials science and surface technology make it possible to control microstructures. Hence it will be possible to produce materials resistant to wear and corrosion, and surface-active biomaterials for forming bonds with tissues for use as implants, and in filter beds and filtration devices.

Progress in microelectronics and in information and communication technology is likely to improve medical information systems and the management of the growing overload of information.

Computer-aided decision-making systems—so-called expert systems—permit the construction of comprehensive libraries of medical records and the use of artificial intelligence.

The rapid growth of technology markets has led in some countries to a certain degree of misuse, apparently a sign of overconsumption of health services. Low-volume, high-cost health technology has been aimed primarily at critical-care medicine and diagnostic technology. However, many countries have not been able to afford to train enough skilled technologists to operate these sophisticated technologies. Also, where insurance coverage is unlimited, high technology uses up an unduly large proportion of health resources, and consequently other social programmes suffer. In countries without general health coverage, health programmes for the poor are cut to satisfy the needs of the insured population.

In developing countries large population groups are denied the benefits of indirect health technologies (sanitation, housing, nutrition, education), and have only very restricted access to direct health technologies in prevention, diagnosis and treatment of diseases. Population growth, urbanization and economic difficulties aggravate this problem. In such circumstances the indiscriminate use of high technology means sophisticated medicine for the few and poor-quality or no care for the great majority.

Nevertheless, the developing countries are under heavy international and internal pressure to import modern medical technology. When they do so, they must then expend scarce resources on buildings, maintenance and staff. Often sophisticated diagnostic procedures are wasted because a country lacks the corresponding therapeutic technologies.

Health-care technologies need to be assessed and regulated, therefore. Assessment should refer to justification of purpose, to quality and to price. Clearly, ways of applying health technology must take account also of how it is transferred. Many health problems can be treated, even prevented, with available, relatively simple and affordable technology.

In many countries, the use of drugs, equipment and other materials in health care is regulated to ensure that only those that meet prescribed standards may be purchased. However, regulation should not stifle innovation or local initiative and research. Standards of quality, safety and efficacy should correspond to countries' needs and level of socioeconomic development.

Technology transfer raises also the issue of intellectual property and patents in connection with new health-technology industries in developing countries.

The question "whose responsibility is health technology transfer?" has a major ethical component. Its answer should be grounded in the universally valid ethical principles of individual autonomy, beneficence and non-maleficence, and distributive justice.

Research has a major role in the development of new technology, and the process of defining and prioritizing research objectives must take account of ethical as well as technical considerations.

Once a technology has advanced from animal laboratories to testing on humans, further issues arise about the involvement of human subjects in assessing its safety and efficacy. Whose standards of research ethics should apply if a technology is developed in one country for use in another? Is it ethical to refuse for any reason, even a moral or religious reason, the transfer of a technology that is unacceptable in the country where it was developed to another country with a compelling need of it? Technologies are not value-free in the moral sense, as *in vitro* fertilization, for instance, has shown. Is it ethical to transfer such technology without regard to the values it bears? Also, the receiver of a technology must weigh the ethical consequences of choosing to receive it.

It was against this very complex background that the Conference entitled Health Technology Transfer — Whose Responsibility? was organized. Its aim was to permit a multidisciplinary group representing the various aspects of health-technology transfer to discuss and determine the roles and responsibilities of the different partners engaged in technology transfer; and to discuss and gain a deeper understanding of the perspectives of both developers and users of health-care technology. The discussions highlighted the gaps between the offer and the need, and suggested means of bridging them. It recognized the different interests of providers and users, and the need for international collaboration.

The conference participants supported a suggestion that, in view of the rapid advances in health technology and the risks associated with its unregulated or indiscriminate transfer to developing countries, WHO, in association with other international organizations concerned with health development in developing countries, should expand and intensify its already influential role in guiding and advising on its transfer. One possible means of doing so would be the establishment under WHO auspices of a task force which would be responsible for, *inter alia*, collating, assessing and disseminating knowledge and information gained from experience in Member States in technology transfer. Such a body could have a number of functions, such as the study of trends and developments in the transfer of all forms of health technology; the correlating and coordination of WHO's activities in technology transfer; cooperation with other concerned international organizations; the sponsorship of promotion of research into the determinants of success and failure in technology transfer, and into methods of evaluating technology; advising on sources of supply of technology, on its effectiveness and cost-efficiency, and on aspects of installation and maintenance; and assisting in assessing needs and priorities in technology transfer in the special circumstances of different countries. The Conference also supported a suggestion that WHO might stimulate or sponsor the establishment of a foundation which would promote and support health technology transfer.

In its concluding session, the Conference emphasized WHO's pivotal and unique role in increasing the effectiveness of health technology transfer, by accepting challenges, offering unbiased opinions, and acting as a repository and facilitator of information transfer.

Zbigniew Bankowski
Secretary-General, CIOMS

OPENING OF THE CONFERENCE

Francisco Vilardell
President, CIOMS

Doctor Nakajima, Director-General of the World Health Organization,
Doctor Murilho Belchior, past President of CIOMS,
Members of the Council for International Organizations of Medical Sciences,
Distinguished Guests,
Ladies and Gentlemen,

As President of CIOMS, it is for me a great privilege to welcome you all to this XXIIIrd CIOMS Round Table Conference, which is organized jointly with the World Health Organization. Its difficult subject "Health Technology Transfer - Whose Responsibility" is most timely. It is easy for all to see that the enormous variation among countries in their geographical, ecological, socioeconomic, political and cultural peculiarities may raise serious ethical and human-value issues. For this reason, CIOMS, as part of its long-term programme on Health Policy, Ethics and Human Values—an International Dialogue, is taking up this theme, following the initiative of the WHO Bi-Regional Conference on Technology Transfer in the Health Field, which was held in Tokyo in 1985.

Of all the moral principles that provide the basis of medical ethics, the most relevant in relation to the subject of this Conference is the principle of justice. Problems of distributive justice arise mostly under conditions of scarcity and competition, particularly when scarce resources are confronted with the inexorable expansion of high-priced, often over-priced, technologies. To many practising physicians, and I am one of them, it has become clear, more and more, that the benefits of high technology, mainly the postponement of death and the lessening of disability, often demand too high a price. The proportion of patients who stand to benefit from high technology follows too often a negative cost-benefit correlation—the more expensive the technique, the fewer the individuals who will be able to profit from it. Not only are there problems in deciding whether to allocate funds for the transfer of a new technology, but also there are problems in allocating the accepted technological advances with fairness. On what principles and policies can equity in the allocation of resources best be achieved? Balancing benefits and burdens of high technology, assessing the cost-effectiveness of their transfer, discussing the problems and opportunities in the transfer of knowledge and analysing factors in the acceptance and appliance of these technologies in countries often ill-prepared to absorb them are some of the topics which, I hope, will be amply discussed during this Conference.

On behalf of CIOMS, may I thank Dr Hiroshi Nakajima, Director-General, for the precious cooperation of the World Health Organization, which co-sponsors this Conference; Professor George Ada, Chairman of the Conference and the members of its Planning Committee; and Professor Zbigniew Bankowski, Secretary-General of CIOMS, for the excellent organization of this meeting. Thank you all for being here.

Dr Hiroshi Nakajima
Director-General, World Health Organization

Mr Chairman,
Mr President,
Distinguished Colleagues and Guests,
Ladies and Gentlemen,

Mr Chairman, may I first say how pleased I am to be here this morning to open this Conference. I should like to welcome you all to Geneva. I trust your stay will be an enlightening and fruitful one. I cannot conceive of any topic that is more relevant to WHO's mission, as we approach the final decade of the twentieth century, than that of this Conference. Hence, it is a source of deep satisfaction to me that WHO has been associated with CIOMS in its planning and organization.

All of us owe a profound debt of gratitude to you, Professor Vilardell, and to you, Dr Bankowski, for your unfailing support of WHO in the many areas that are crucial to its constitutional mandate, but which a body such as CIOMS is perhaps better suited to address than WHO itself. I am particularly pleased and encouraged by the development of the CIOMS programme "Health Policy, Ethics and Human Values — An International Dialogue". The classification and resolution of ethical issues are of vital importance to the advancement of public health, and yet this is a field in which an intergovernmental organization such as WHO has to tread very varily. We benefit enormously therefore from the efforts of CIOMS to exchange information, experience and insight in such areas as human experimentation, experiments on animals, family planning, the mapping of the human genome, and—the topic of the present conference—the basic ethical issues implicit in the transfer of technology and of intellectual property.

WHO's Constitution does not give specific and detailed guidance on health technology; yet the subject permeates all the functions outlined in Article 2, and we do have a mandate to work in this field, a mandate which we have not neglected, and which I intend to strengthen in my term of office as Director-General. Let me remind you, in particular, that in May 1976 the World Health Assembly adopted Resolution WHA29.74, in which it indicated its desire for WHO's activities in the field of health technology to be strengthened. Subsequent resolutions, adopted in May 1980 and May 1986, placed further emphasis on health care technology. Also, we find a strong emphasis on health technology and its transfer in the historic Declaration of Alma-Ata, adopted in September 1978.

Time does not permit me to dwell in detail on the manifold activities related to technology in which we are currently engaged. They include vigorous programmes on the technologies of health laboratories, blood transfusion and related activities, radiology, clinical medicine and rehabilitation. We place emphasis not merely on technology itself but also on its transfer, particularly to and among developing countries. In a few of the WHO regions, there is vigorous dialogue and discussion about the

2

ways and means of transferring technology. Mr President, you have already mentioned one meeting which I organized with my colleagues in the Western Pacific Region a few years ago. This provided guidance to some extent, but since then of course there have been further developments. The transfer of intellectual property has been raised in GATT (General Agreement on Tariffs and Trade) recently, encountering opposition from a few industrialized countries. I believe the discussions in GATT are continuing. In fact this raises the basic issue of the right of every man and woman to have access to, at least, essential technology or to the technology available, such as essential drugs. You know that in some industrialized countries the ever-increasing cost of some technology has made some governments decide not to make it available to certain population groups. So these ethical issues raised by technology transfer are becoming more pertinent in discussions on public health, since they indicate conflict between the basic human right of every individual and the collective right to health. This may become a wider issue in the future. I believe that CIOMS is a much more suitable forum than WHO in which to talk freely on this kind of issue. I listened with much pleasure to the speech of Professor John H. Bryant at the 1989 Gala Dinner of the Medical Society of WHO, on the occasion of the 40th anniversary of CIOMS; also, I am glad that CIOMS is organizing a conference on *Genetics, ethics and human values: human genome mapping, genetic screening and genetic therapy,* in Tokyo and Inuyama City in July 1990.

Ladies and Gentlemen, I am looking forward with great interest to the results of your Conference. Its outcome will help to guide me in the decisions I shall be taking shortly to strengthen and consolidate our programmes in this area, particularly the development of health technology. The title of the Conference ends with a question mark. As far as WHO is concerned, the answer to the question is resoundingly positive. Under our Constitution, WHO is responsible for acting as the directing and coordinating authority in international health work. We intend to exercise that responsibility to the full in the field of health-technology transfer. In doing so, we shall rely on the cooperation and support of our partners inside and outside the United Nations system, and of our colleagues and friends in such organizations as CIOMS. We are entering a period where discussions among all involved, on appropriate technology and the "appropriation" of technology, and even the assessment of technology for transfer, may be the first step towards the transfer of technology among countries, and especially between industrialized and developing countries.

Professor Vilardell and Dr Bankowski, I am confident that this Conference will be as successful as its predecessors, some of which I have been privileged to attend. Your Chairman, Professor Ada, has long experience in this field in the Western Pacific Region, as well as in WHO meetings on the subject; his able guidance is sure to be most appreciated and will surely bring positive results.

3

HIGHLIGHTS OF THE CONFERENCE

Gordon Ada*

Introduction

Technology has been defined as the body of tools emerging from the interplay of scientific knowledge and practical operation applied to specialized services. When applied to the health area, the term includes medical/scientific technology, equipment-embodied technology and ancillary technology. Health technology transfer (HTT) is the transfer of such technology from one group or organization within a country (or internationally) to another group within the same or a different country. HTT occurs at different levels. Though many would consider that transfer of information, knowledge, scientific techniques and industrial processes are major features, transfer of the "fruits"of technology, say marketing a drug, may have indirect benefits such as marketing experience, which might lead later to the local development of the technology, such as the production of the drug or other drugs.

HTT has been and remains a major component of WHO's activities, as is seen in the work of several of the Divisions of the Organization. This varies from the establishment of lists of appropriate equipment in selected areas, the provision of specifications for equipment of simplified but effective design, and the selection of centres where there is experience in the design and fabrication of medical equipment, to the activities of the two Special Programmes, for Research and Training in Tropical Diseases, and of Research, Development and Research Training in Human Reproduction. These programmes have segments directed to strengthening of research capability of institutes and groups in the developing countries.

It was becoming increasingly clear some years ago that application of the newer technologies arising from concepts in the biological and physical sciences would have a major impact on the research carried out under the auspices of the Special Programmes. An awareness of the potential of these advances in technology to contribute to the work of not only the Special Programmes but also other WHO programmes led the Global Advisory Committee of Medical Research in 1983 to establish a subcommittee to study and report on "The enhancement of transfer of technology to developing countries with special reference to health". The subcommittee produced a report (WHO/ROD/ACHR/(TT)/87) which was presented to the annual meeting in 1986 of the Global Advisory Committee of Health Research (as it had then been named). The report was distributed widely, comments were received and a final document and responses to it were discussed at the 29th Session of the Advisory Committee in 1988.

---

* Professor, The John Curtin School of Medical Research, Canberra, Australia.

A major charge of the subcommittee was to review the recent advances in the biological and physical sciences and to assess the impact these might have in the health area if the technology concerned could be transferred to developing countries. The factors that affect the success of HTT were also considered and several proposals were made which might contribute to solving some of the perceived problems and difficulties.

In further recognition of the importance of this topic the Council for International Organizations of Medical Sciences (CIOMS) convened its XXIIIrd Round Table Conference to discuss the question—Health Technology Transfer - Whose Responsibility? It was organized jointly with WHO, particularly with the Office of Research Promotion and Development and the Division of Diagnostics, Therapeutics and Rehabilitation Technology. The invited speakers and those in the audience represented a wide range of disciplines and came from many countries.

Despite often the best intentions and the availability of technology for transfer, there continue to be many examples of inappropriate transfer, particularly of specialized, high-cost equipment which remains unused, or used for short periods only before a breakdown occurs, and repairs cannot be made locally. Examples are quoted of "major disaster areas", where factories have been constructed without all the necessary experience and specialized knowledge required for their operation and maintenance. A major aim of this conference was to identify some of the critical factors that contribute to successful transfer and to consider how they can be incorporated into transfer programmes.

The Director-General of WHO, Dr Hiroshi Nakajima, opened the conference and re-affirmed not only that HTT would remain a priority subject for WHO but also that it was intended to extend WHO's activities in this direction and that the matter was under discussion. His presentation set the stage for what developed into a lively and productive meeting.

The programme was divided into three parts—Trends in Technology Transfer; Partners in Technology Transfer, from the perspectives of both developed and developing countries; and the Role of Facilitators of Technology Transfer.

Trends in Technology Transfer

New developments in high technology
The last two decades have witnessed a remarkable burgeoning of high-performance (and costly) medical devices based on advances in the physical sciences. These are very largely devoted to improving the quality and sensitivity of diagnostic tests, and improving therapy, and to supportive and ameliorative procedures. Computerized tomography (CT), positron emission tomography (PET) and nuclear magnetic resonance imaging (MRI) are but a few. Many of these developments would have been impossible without the availability of computers or their equivalent.

5

Compared with other developments, computer technology has been almost unique in that cost has been steadily reduced and quality improved. Many of these techniques are still being explored for their applicability; for example, it has been reported that only about 20% of all patients who presently undergo CT scanning obtain any benefit from it.

Advances in the biological techniques have been equally impressive. The ability to manipulate DNA, to clone cells, to prepare chemically pure preparations of biologically active proteins, including antibodies of a single specificity, not only has had a profound effect on the pace of research but also is beginning to have clinical and industrial impact. For example, the first vaccine made by yeast cells transfected with DNA coding for the surface antigen (HBsAg) of hepatitis B virus is now on the market.

Assessment of effectiveness of HTT
Health technology (HT) innovation in developed countries, such as the USA, is directed mainly towards the individual rather than the community. It has been estimated that 50% of spending for acute medical services in the USA is on behalf of only 4% of the patient population. The cost of HT varies greatly, from an estimated $ 2 000 per head in the USA to about $ 2 per head in rural areas of some developing countries. Few countries have established mechanisms for the systematic evaluation of new medical knowledge and technology, except for the products of the drug industry. Optimally, health-care services should be adjusted and matched to socially and professionally determined needs, but more often than not their content and form are determined by the providers in an atmosphere of competition, covert advertisement and public-relations practices.

Few countries have developed comprehensive prevention programmes, including better nutrition, housing, intervention in unhealthy lifestyles (smoking and alcohol abuse), health education, immunization and sanitation.

Ethical aspects of HTT
The question—whose responsibility? has a major ethical component. The three central values—beneficence, autonomy and justice—emerged from an interaction of physicians with society, but related mainly to individual patients. In HTT the power lies with firms and governments rather than with the medical fraternity. Will questions be asked, such as—what types of knowledge will be sought? and, towards ameliorating what disease, eg., infectious diseases compared with cancer? Whose standards of research ethics should apply if a technology is developed in country A for use in country B? Is it appropriate for a country to refuse, for any reason including moral or religious objections, the transfer of a technology that is unacceptable domestically to another country whose need for that technology is very great? Is it ethical for the values attached to the technology also to be transferred with the technology? It may be impossible to avoid such issues arising; the receiver of the technology must weigh the ethical consequences when making the choice to receive it.

Problems and opportunities in the transfer of knowledge
Of all the factors that influence the priorities of choice in HTT in the receiving country, the availability of resources and infrastructure to make the transferred technology viable in the user country is the most imponderable. Expectations must be realistic. There must be a "critical mass" of professionals with specific capabilities, and this includes an informed understanding of the basic science underlying the technology. This latter point is critical, for technology never stands still. Technicians must be trained in a range of skills. An educational system, both school and university, which encourages enquiring minds is essential, particularly for design and synthesis.

One approach to achieving this is the use of artificial-intelligence techniques to facilitate the teaching process. The relevant knowledge required to achieve a successful transfer can be incorporated into a computer-based "expert consultative system", assembled by the provider and used as an adjunct to normal transfer procedures.

Problems and opportunities in the absorption of technology
As seen from the viewpoint of a user country, five issues are of paramount importance. They are:

- the need for a national health care policy—what technologies are needed, for what purpose and at what level of health care?
- receptor mechanisms for absorption of technology—the infrastructure necessary to absorb the transferred technology;
- an adequate information system—the need to make the right choices in choosing technology for transfer;
- research and development units—needed to facilitate transfer and to foster comparable indigenous technologies;
- fostering a culture in which the importance of science and technology is appreciated and encouraged.

Roles of regulatory authories
There is a need to assess the safety and efficacy of medical devices. Manufacturers or sponsors should register their products, comply with labelling requirements and generally follow Good Manufacturing Practices. Information supplied by a manufacturer often needs to be reviewed by other experts, not only for verification but also for suitability for transfer to other groups or for use for purposes other than the original description.

Even within developed countries, and far more so in developing countries, there is a great need of mechanisms for exchanging such information. This is particularly so if a device manufactured in one country proves, for one reason or another, to be faulty in the same or a different country. To carry out such duties effectively, an international network needs to be established. Once this is achieved, the difficulties in implementing regulations can be resolved more effectively than at present.

7

Partners in Technology Transfer: the Perspective of Industrialized Countries

Technical cooperation agencies
The guiding principle of such agencies is to act only at the request of recipient governments. The health budgets of provider governments is small and therefore competition for available funds is great. In recent years, the emphasis has switched to primary health care, but in this area there are sensitive issues such as family planning, which is desperately needed in many countries.

Implementation of HTT is often difficult. Suitable technologies are often readily available but there is not the capacity to absorb them. Sometimes the great variety of technologies donated to a country compounds the difficulty because they cannot be serviced or maintained. Few developing countries have the capacity to produce drugs and control their quality. With such diseases as AIDS on the increase, a high proportion of the scarce resources are now being devoted to diagnostic facilities.

The dilemma facing provision of health technology is that there are too many pressure groups, on both the provider and the user sides. To be equitable, assistance should be limited to life-saving technologies for all, but generally this is politically and culturally unacceptable. Tourism is often a valuable source of foreign exchange and tourists demand high-tech health facilities. Thus, a high proportion of available resources support tertiary-care hospitals, which benefit a minority of the local population, while the majority suffer from a lack of basic medical services.

The Pharmaceutical Industry
For the main reason that medicines and vaccines are and will be, at least in the near future, the main arm in the control of disease in both developing and developed countries, the role of the pharmaceutical industry in health technology transfer should not be underestimated. New technology will almost certainly continue to be created in industrialized countries and subsequently transferred to developing countries.

The range of technology will extend from the drug product itself, which should be regarded as being inseparable from the information on its therapeutic indications and proper use, at one end of the spectrum, to technical expertise in the manufacture of intermediates for the drug substance, at the other end. It will include information which has been generated to establish its safety, quality and efficacy, expert knowledge on the manufacture of drug substance, formulation, packaging, plant design and construction, and, most important, tests methods and quality-control procedures.

Universities
Many of the basic teaching skills needed to train personnel to understand and maintain medical devices can be effectively carried out in a university environment if the teaching programme is planned well in advance. A major limitation to the success of the transfer is the support available

8

when trainees return to their own countries. The transfer process itself is best done by personnel who understand the basic scientific principles and possess tact, experience and patience.

Frequently the actual transfer is not clear-cut. There is sometimes frank deception about a device by a provider, equipment may be wrongly labelled, and too often the transferred equipment is unnecessarily high-tech: a simple X-ray machine will benefit far more people than a CT. In addition, prices are sometimes kept artificially high by a manufacturer.

Universities, like WHO, have an important and perhaps a unique role. They should teach attitudes, not merely techniques. They can give a dispassionate assessment of such aspects as cost/benefit. Above all, knowledge must be transferred freely and openly. Often however, commercial aspects take precedence, and this may raise difficulties. How should a university react if it is clear that a decision taken is not the best for the whole community? Should it wait to be asked for advice or take active steps? Universities, like WHO, should be prepared to give guidance.

Research and service institutions
Ideally, these institutions should be in a good position to play an effective role in HTT. They have well-trained staff who are experienced in handling a variety of complex medical devices. They sometimes establish links with a counterpart institute in a user country. They could help in many ways, but particularly in staff training in the technology most appropriate for the needs of the developing country. In reality, as research and service institutions were not established for this purpose, they have generally found it difficult to find the necessary resources—funds, personnel etc—to do an effective job. They can make, and are making, a modest contribution, which is most helpful if both the institute and the recipient plan well in advance and agree on a specific type of technology—one of which the institute has expert knowledge and experience and which is most suited to the needs of the user country.

Partners in Technology Transfer: the Perspective of Developing Countries

Economists
The most important economic message is that the economic progress of a developing country depends upon receiving appropriate technology transfer. The first objective is to utilize the relatively more abundant resources to improve labour and/or capital productivity for economic growth. A country must be able to absorb the transferred technology, and to have the technological capability and socio-economic infrastructure to develop its own technology, based on the imported kind. In contrast to many other forms of technology, HTT can directly improve a country's *human* capital, both quantitatively and qualitatively. It improves the quality of labour and production efficiency.

9

It has recently been recognized that a major factor contributing to the success of recently industrialized economies can be attributed to investment in human capital—in education and in health. Both lay the foundation for sustained increase in labour productivity. For an economist the issue becomes a matter of prioritizing "investment options" in human health. This includes both indirect (housing, sanitation etc) and direct HTT.

Usually, HTT means Western-country-type medical care. Many developing countries (e.g., in the Orient) have indigenous practices, and care should be taken to have an appropriate mix of technologies. There should not be aggressive sales campaigns, e.g., cigarettes, baby foods, unless there is clear evidence of the benefits of the technology, as would be the case with vaccines. The transfer should not result in dependency on the provider country; rather, it should exert a positive influence on the trading ability of the user country. Once a user country reaches a critical mass of high-quality human capital, it reaches a "take-off point" on the road to economic growth, which in turn makes more realistic the goal of "health for all by the year 2000".

Health ministries
The health systems inherited by many countries from colonial powers after the Second World War were biased towards large hospitals and curative services. Mortality rates decreased but there was little influence on morbidity, especially in vulnerable groups such as mothers and young children. Adjustments made over the years in developing countries were aimed at providing more comprehensive health care, focusing on health promotion and prevention of ill-health. A few countries have made very commendable advances in this direction.

A number of action areas have been identified which would hasten the achievement of these goals. They include intensifying community involvement, leadership development, interaction between different sectors, strengthening of different health systems and manpower development.

Universities
How does a developing country decide between high technology for the few and basic medical services for the many—between the exciting advances in the medical-devices area, in knowledge and understanding, and the basic needs such as complete immunization coverage, good diagnosis and simple but effective medical devices? The Third-World university is in a unique position to help to resolve this problem. Though it may be inadequately funded and staffed, it can develop strong links with universities in First World countries and so have access to many of the new developments, and at the same time be conscious of the conditions and needs of the population as a whole.

The three main functions of a university—education, service and research—can help bridge the gaps, particularly if a partnership with government can be forged. Formulation of a national health policy is a first step, and its implementation will address those deficiencies in the existing system. Cost-effectiveness analysis can determine the appropriateness of different alternatives—lithotripsy or growth monitoring, tuberculosis control or intensive neonatal-care units, etc. These decisions raise serious ethical questions, which must be squarely faced if an equitable health system is to be fashioned.

Infrastructure and manpower
These two aspects are at the heart of the needs of a user country if it is to be able to absorb HTT. A variety of unfortunate but common practices contribute greatly to the wastage of limited national resources. To overcome these major obstacles, four courses of action are indicated:

1. The formulation and implementation of an organizational policy. This may result in the formulation of a national health policy, which can be advertised at awareness seminars for workers at different levels. This may be aided by the establishment of a "standing policy and planning committee".
2. The development of an effective system of health-care technical services (HCTS) providing a high standard of service. Its functions would include the proper selection, specification and procurement of equipment, planning, inventory control, routine preventive maintenance and repairs, and training of staff. The system should be available to both urban and rural hospitals and health units.
3. Adequate manpower development and training of staff at all levels of the health sector. This includes attractive career structures and salaries. The formation of national training centres and regional international centres greatly facilitates this process; WHO can help greatly with the latter.
4. In most countries, a substantial improvement of the means of collecting, collating, assessing, disseminating and updating technical information. The variety and ready accessibility of computer-based programmes using comprehensive data-banks facilitate this process.

A few developing countries, sometimes with WHO help, have made great progress in implementing such programmes and may serve as a source of information and an example for other countries.

Facilitators of Health Technology Transfer

International organizations
WHO has already made notable contributions in this area, but an analysis of major constraints suggests additional approaches that WHO and sister organizations can assist in developing. Some requirements are paramount. The first is the political will of the country to establish the infrastructure for the effective absorption of HTT. A second is the availability of sufficient human resources to assemble a coherent picture of national needs. A third is the recognition that a process of selection and exclusion is necessary. There are opportunities here to develop new or improved methods of determining and ranking priorities and allocating resources. Time becomes a critical factor. All effort should not be

placed on short-term goals—a balance should be reached between short- and long-term goals.

To cope with such problems, better planning methods and tools are required. Ranking priorities on a rational basis, for example, can be achieved only if the complex interrelationships of various health problems and other socioeconomic problems are understood. Only too often, interventions to achieve health development may have major effects outside the health sector, and vice versa. The costs and consequences of intended strategies within and outside the health sector must be appreciated. New methods, new information and new insights are needed, and WHO sees a responsibility for itself in promoting the research necessary to develop the new methodologies.

How may this be achieved? One step would be to broaden the spectrum of scientific advice available to WHO, a recommendation already made by its Advisory Committee of Health Research. An advisory group for this purpose would operate flexibly to monitor and forecast new scientific and technological developments. A second step would be to strengthen the relationship between WHO and scientific institutions, world-wide, particularly regarding problem-related issues. A third would be to gain the capacity to forecast new, relevant technological developments. HTT should be concerned with not only goods and productive capacity but also the capacity to think and to innovate. The success rate of HTT would undoubtedly increase if these approaches could be widely implemented.

Forecasters
Industrialized countries often have mechanisms in both government and industry to translate the findings of biomedical and physical scientific research into technology. This is increasingly being accompanied by an emphasis on both the safety and the efficacy of the new technology, and this is the case with health-care technology.

It is a hazardous undertaking to attempt to forecast new scientific developments—those advances that may win for the discoverer the highest academic recognition. But it is possible and feasible to look back for a variable time, say 5–15 years, to assess the progress made in a particular area in the application of scientific findings to technology development and to forecast the extent to which these developments will continue and expand in the future. Such forecasting has obvious implications for HTT if a user country is to gain the most benefit in the long term from a transferred technology.

There have been many spectacular advances in both the biological and the physical sciences. The ability to manipulate DNA, in particular, has revolutionized several disciplines, notably genetics and immunology, and similar effects, such as information processing, have followed discoveries in the physical sciences. How can long-term development in health-care technology from such advances be assessed? In a recent study commissioned by the Government of the Netherlands the opinions of hundreds of experts were surveyed, and in a follow-up some were selected for in-depth study. These included neurosciences—the regeneration of nervous tissue, lasers—treatment of coronary heart disease, and biotechnology—new vaccines, to name a few. It was concluded that a system needs to be established for monitoring research developments and their possible influence on health care. This would be best achieved through international collaboration, based on a number of focal points. WHO could have a critical role in such a scenario.

Technology brokers

The traditional and still widely used approach between countries has been for the government of the provider country to identify the need for certain skills in a developing country, and to send an expert to give a training programme, following which the parties frequently separated. The failure rate of this approach has been substantial. Some significant transfers were made to developing countries by subsidiaries of transnational corporations. However, objections were often raised about foreign firms seeking equity investments or licensing arrangements for their industrial property, which led to restrictions on such joint ventures. More recently, enterprise-to-enterprise transfer is being seen as perhaps a more realistic and effective way to accelerate the industrial development of the Third World. Some developing countries are now moving to facilitate the transfer to local firms of a wide range of production technologies deemed important for their development.

This trend has led to the establishment in Geneva of the organization "Technology for the People" (TFTP), which seeks contracts from donor countries or agencies to directly support technology transfer and international trade on a company-to-company basis, with an element of profit as the driving force. TFTP and similar consulting organizations now serve the interests mainly of small to medium-sized companies that are willing to offer their technology and know-how to Third World firms. This occurs not only from North to South but also from South to South. Experience over the last few years illustrates the skills and attitudes needed by a successful technology broker. The include the ability and willingness:

- to identify and cultivate potential clients;
- to generate credibility and trust among prospective clients;
- to sort through and select the relevant information;
- to invest time in building up company contracts and information sources; and
- to provide information about sources of financial assistance.

Besides bringing the parties together and creating an environment conducive to success, patience and fortitude to "see it through" are necessary characteristics.

Independent consultants

Technology transfer between the most technically rich country, the provider or *reservoir,* and the least technically rich country, the user or *potential,* is often regarded as the most desirable scenario. From the potential user's point of view, there is direct access to the most advanced

13

capabilities, and for the provider/reservoir there may be a large and now accessible market. However, there are many advantages in a two-stage process in which the reservoir country transfers technology to a country with an intermediate status—a *transceiver* country. Such a country possesses sufficient skills in the various important categories—management, design capability, documentation at a suitable level, manufacturing experience and a distribution network—to greatly enhance the prospect of success of the transfer. Such countries can often provide suitable substitute materials etc, and thus limit the need to import high-tech (and expensive) materials and equipment.

The transceiver country, in turn, appreciates more the true needs and difficulties of the final-user country, as it may well have been in this category previously. There will also be substantially lower costs all round, but particularly in manpower and materials. The technology may be modified to allow a more labour-intensive component to utilize existing strengths of the user-country.

In either situation, the consultant can have a direct or indirect role. In the former, the consultant provides the capabilities which both partner countries lack. In this situation, there are great opportunities to offer a wide variety of skills so that otherwise "missing" components are provided, thus enhancing the chances of success. In the latter case, the consultant's role resembles more the broker's, as described previously.

Other examples of facilitation
WHO collaborating centres can make important contributions to HTT. As an example, the work of ECRI, a non-profit, non-governmental agency in Philadelphia, U.S.A., for information transfer on medical devices, was described. It operates an international reporting network to hospitals and health agencies in 45 countries, from the simplest disposable products to the most complex computerized imaging systems. Information is provided in five ways—by publications (> 30 journals), direct consultations and seminars, comparative reports on products, problems and recalls, data-bases on medical-product evaluation, and provision of fellowships (from months to years in length). As a WHO collaborating centre, the organization serves as a world-wide gathering-point for all types of information on medical technology, including the evaluation, organization and dissemination of the information.

At a very different level, the expansion of clinical immunology services since 1975 in a single country, Venezuela, was described. Ten regional clinical-immunology units have been established in that time, servicing about 20 million inhabitants. The success of this venture has depended upon regionalization—individual unit autonomy—and mutual trust between units. This has been a success story of technology transfer within a country.

General Discussion

Technology transfer is as old as mankind. Our ancestor who first found that fire could be generated by friction, by vigorously rubbing two sticks together, and so enabled his tribe to become independent of lightning-strikes for this technology, was in a commanding position to negotiate a favourable trade arrangement with less fortunate tribes. Many volumes have been written on the subject in recent years. What did this conference achieved which will enhance successful HTT?

First of all, there was a remarkable degree of consensus about the complexity of the issues, which must be recognized and taken into account by all parties if HTT is to be successful—to benefit both provider and user. Whether the particular project under consideration qualifies as HTT at the high-tech level or at a village level, sufficient is now known about the ways *not* to go about the transfer. It should be possible now to elaborate guiding principles, which, if adopted, should do much to facilitate HTT. The question of deciding between "high-tech" and "low-tech" transfer—on the one hand to favour the privileged few, including tourists, and, on the other, to provide basic services such as immunization coverage and equipment such as simple X-ray devices—may also appear to be relatively straightforward in principle but is much more complicated and difficult in practice. Such matters are not decided by health experts, apart from the occasional opportunity afforded by a health professional relationship with an influential politician or decision-maker. Political and other considerations are often deciding factors.

The meeting was particularly heartened by the opening remarks of the Director-General of WHO, Dr Nakajima, that WHO not only recognized the importance of its current activities in relation to HTT but also was actively exploring a proposal that this activity be expanded, perhaps by the formation of a special group for this purpose. The thoughtful contribution by the Deputy Director-General, Dr Abdelmoumene, on fundamental aspects of the process of technology transfer was further evidence of the Organization's commitment to such an expansion. Should this take the form of a special group, such as a task force, the opinion was expressed that many of the points raised at the meeting might form part of the initial agenda for consideration. Moreover, some of the participants of the meeting might be able to contribute usefully to this work.

A particularly stimulating session contained presentations on different approaches to facilitating HTT. Several speakers expressed the view that, despite the important role of such international bodies as WHO, there was room for other bodies to act as an interface between the producer and the public sector. One quoted need was to get important products, e.g. in regard to human reproduction, to the public in some countries. Another possibility raised was the establishment of an international body which would provide venture capital to strengthen the private sector in developing countries. Such a fund could facilitate enterprise-to-enterprise ventures, which now seem to be an effective form of HTT, and one which avoids the difficulties often experienced with government-to-government arrangements.

There was general support for a proposal that, in view of the rapid advances in health technology and the risks associated with its indiscriminate transfer to user contries, which were highlighted at this Conference,

WHO should expand its already influential role in advising and assisting on the transfer of health technology to developing countries. One approriate approach would be the establishment, under WHO auspices, of a task force with a number of functions. These would include the study of trends and developments in the transfer of all forms of health technology; the correlation and coordination of WHO's activities in health technology transfer; cooperation with other concerned international organizations; the promotion of research into known and probable determinants of success and failure in technology transfer and into methods of evaluating technology; advising on sources of supply of health technology, on its effectiveness and cost-efficiency, and on aspects of installation and maintenance of equipment; and assisting in assessing the needs and priorities in technology transfer for user countries. To be maximally effective, such a task force should collate, assess and disseminate widely the conclusions and recommendations resulting from consideration of the information from the studies and activities of the task force, together with specific knowledge gained from the experience of WHO's Member States in health technology transfer.

It was suggested also that, as an additional aid, WHO should sponsor the establishment of a foundation which would promote and support health technology transfer.

The Conference re-emphasized WHO's pivotal and unique role in all these aspects of health technology transfer.

TRENDS IN TECHNOLOGY TRANSFER

CURRENT TRENDS IN HIGH TECHNOLOGY

Murray Eden*

It is common knowledge that health-related technologies in many different forms—information processing systems, elaborate diagnostic instruments, new modes of therapy—are playing an increasing role in the delivery of health care in the United States of America and other industrialized countries. Technology has played a very small role in health care until quite recently. The influx of technology followed the commercial introduction of electronics and research for addressing the needs of World War II. Devices originally used for physical and chemical research entered biological research laboratories and, subsequently, the medical milieu.

The tools of physical science tend to be costly, complex to use, and frequently without obvious application to health problems; nevertheless, the opportunity to convert them for use in the health sector aroused the enthusiasm of innovative engineers, physicians and entrepreneurs. In large measure this remains true. The success of a technological innovation in health care requires contributions from a number of parties: inventors, physicians, manufacturers, patients and their families, health care administrators and health ministries. These parties have some interests in common, but they have different requirements, expectations and priorities for the design, applications and mode of operation of medical devices. Moreover, economic, cultural and political realities will constrain or guide the introduction of new technology.

Health technology innovation in the United States, and in other developed countries, is devoted overwhelmingly to improving the quality of diagnosis, therapy and supportive and ameliorative procedures, all directed to the particular needs of individuals. Americans are very much aware of the costs of their health care system, but there is no consensus as to causes of, or steps to remedy, inequities arising from these costs in the delivery of health care. Moreover, while there is a growing recognition of the need for cost containment, the major emphasis is still on improvement of quality and on convenience.

Machine computation stands out as the technology with the most profound effect on the forms that medical devices and systems have taken. Digital electronics, microprocessors and computers are indispensable in high-technology devices, including medical devices.

---

* National Institutes of Health, Division of Research Services, Biomedical Engineering and Instrumentation Branch, Bethesda, MD, USA.

This work was performed by the author as part of his employment by the Government of the United States. The opinions expressed in this paper are solely those of the author and do not necessarily reflect official DHHS opinion.

The influence of electronic advances upon biomedical instrumentation is not purely economic. True, less costly electronics may lead to less expensive devices that use them, but, more important, progress in microcircuits technology can lead to fundamental changes in the design of medical devices, including expanding their use within the framework of diagnosis and extending their application from diagnosis to the control of therapy.

Computers are indispensable components of the high-technology devices of biological research and medical practice, especially imaging devices. Computerized tomography (CT), positron emission tomography (PET), nuclear magnetic resonance imaging (MRI)—indeed all medical imaging technologies developed since CT—would be utterly impractical if their numerical computation had to be done by hand. This is as true of ultrasound imaging as it is of PET imaging, although the computer is an ultrasound imager and by no means as visible (or as expensive) as the image in the PET scanner. What is not commonly appreciated is that there is a computer or its equivalent in virtually every modern product of medical instrument technology. Personal computers, microprocessors and the other modules they require—printers, displays, memories—are relatively inexpensive. Component development and commercial competition have maintained low costs, whereas reliability has increased and microprocessors have become more powerful. Currently, the major costs are incurred in programming rather than in hardware. An increasing number of specialty programs have been written and are commercially available for many different health-related tasks, such as record keeping, scheduling, diagnostic assistance, and archiving of pictures. Networking of health-related data has also developed rapidly and will use the many advances in communications technology, including improved satellite transmission, fiber optic cables, etc. Parallel processors and supercomputers are still largely research tools, but important uses are being found in the pharmaceutical industry for drug design.

Biological laboratories and commercial enterprises are continuing the development of imaging devices. The current state of clinical diagnostic radiology has been summarized by Alexander Margulis, Chief of Radiology at the University of California at San Francisco, and a pioneer in the use of magnetic resonance imaging[1].

"Radiology has benefitted from the explosive growth of imaging technology. During the last 10 years several new cross-sectional imaging modalities have appeared, considerably improving the sensitivity of radiologic diagnosis and in many instances also improving the specificity. The new imaging modalities, ultrasound with the newest addition, color doppler, computed tomography and magnetic resonance imaging and spectroscopy are revolutionizing the field.

"Even conventional radiography has undergone significant change with the development of the double contrast examination, particularly of the esophagus, stomach and colon, which has significantly improved the detection of small neoplastic lesions. The introduction of enteroclysis has made a diagnosis of small bowel abnormalities considerably more precise and has made detection of even small lesions a reality.

"Ultrasound and computed tomography in addition to adding information about abnormalities in the abdomen and staging of various types of cancer have also allowed the guidance of needle biopsy which in turn has made preoperative histologic or microbiologic diagnosis a reality and eliminated to a great extent exploratory laparotomies.

"Ultrasonography has become the true imaging screening approach. There is today a spectrum of devices from very inexpensive and relatively unsophisticated that are used as part of the physical examination complementing the stethoscope to extremely sophisticated devices that are digital and also contain color doppler. In addition to these devices there are also more invasive approaches like intraoperative ultrasound, transrectal, transvaginal probes and transducers connected with endoscopes.

"Computed tomography is rapidly replacing conventional radiology as the screening imaging device. Computed tomography is so versatile that it is being applied throughout the body and has totally replaced conventional tomography of the lungs, and many barium studies of the bowel. An important new application of computed tomography is the determination of calcification in coronary arteries on millisecond scans. The significance of coronary calcification is much greater in the fourth, fifth, and sixth decades of life than in the seventh or later. With computed tomography becoming one of the main imaging methods, a whole spectrum of machines has been developed by industry.

"Magnetic resonance has become an indispensable diagnostic tool in modern diagnosis. Its greatest advantages are in increased soft tissue contrast resolution and in the possibility of direct imaging in any imaging plane. Individualization of technique which has greatly increased the sensitivity of the method is due to the presence of seven imaging parameters—proton density, T1 and T2 relaxation parameters, proton, bulk motion, chemical shift, diffusion constant and magnetic susceptibility.

"MR has become indispensable for the diagnosis of afflictions of the brain, spinal cord, male and female pelvis and the musculoskeletal system including the spine. MR is also equal to or better than other imaging approaches in the diagnosis of abnormalities of the face, neck, heart, and mediastinum. It is also very good in the liver and approaches are being developed for the diagnosis of abnormalities of the spleen. Multiple machines are being developed from those with permanent magnets with very low magnetic field strength, 0.03 to 0.06, to sophisticated high-field devices of 1.5 to 2.0 Tesla. Techniques replacing angiography and assessing and measuring flow are being developed. Improvements are occurring also in spatial resolution, in the speed of scanning, in sensitivity and also in specificity. For improvement in specificity, contrast media, computer approaches, localized tissue spectroscopy and chemical shift imaging are being introduced, as well as magnetic susceptibility and diffusion imaging."

21

Imaging technology, especially MRI, is being rapidly developed. MRI is costly, but it is also a powerful diagnostic tool. Its development is almost entirely in commercial hands. Research has concentrated on improving resolution, shortening imaging time and exploring labelling techniques for the detection of tumors and other pathologies. A recently developed MRI technique permits the imaging of thermal gradients *in vivo* and its use in hyperthermia is being studied. NMR spectroscopy is still a research tool but may ultimately be useful in identifying physiological malfunction. Fine-structure proton and phosphorus spectra can be obtained *in vivo* from arbitrary volumes in the body as small as 1 cm^3.

CT scanners have been available for about 15 years and have had considerable commercial success, but they are now regarded as having significant limitations. Today's conventional CT scanners have scan speeds of 1–4 seconds and spatial resolution of 0.5–1.0 mm, and sell for a cost of 0.5–1.0 million dollars. Thus conventional CT is slower, has less resolution, and is more expensive than many other X-ray procedures. A CT chest study will provide a wealth of diagnostic information compared to a chest film, but the use of an expensive CT scanner for about one hour makes this type of examination impractical.

New CT scanner technology addresses many of these limitations. Ultrafast electron-beam-based systems offer scan speeds in the 60 millisecond range. An electron-beam-based Ultrafast CT scanner (FAS-TRAC^{TM} Picker) can perform a chest CT study in one minute of scanning and an additional six minutes of processing for 40 levels. In the next few years this type of study will be further reduced in cost and the number of levels increased. Higher resolution scanners with image matrices of 1024×1024 picture elements will become available soon. Improved high-voltage designs, newer high-speed microcomputer designs, and the replacement of mechanical motion with a scanned electron beam have made these developments possible.

Two new approaches to positron emission tomography (PET) are being studied. The first approach is the traditional one, which seeks higher resolution and higher sensitivity imaging by using a more advanced multidetector array such as a multilayer cylindrical or spherical system. This approach has been the mainstream of the recent PET developments and has helped the development of several new high-stopping-power detectors such as BGO and GSO. Further developments along this line include the various image reconstruction algorithms associated with the system, such as 3-D image reconstruction algorithms and iterative algorithms based on statistical models.

Another direction of PET design, simple and likely to be more cost-effective, is a resolution system suitable for certain specific applications, such as brain imaging. It achieves these benefits by concentrating the imaging analysis of small volumes. This design, which is still under development, is claimed to permit an affordable, highly-efficient, reliable high-resolution PET system, useful for physiological studies of the brain that require extremely high resolution within a limited region.

In neurology, PET is being used to study cerebral, metabolic and hemodynamic dysfunctions that occur as a result of pathological processes affecting the brain. These include studies of alterations in flow and metabolism, the cerebral autoregulatory response, metabolic substrate utilization and effects of ischemia. While still only a research tool, it may ultimately have predictive value for patients at risk from stroke.

Imaging at the level of the cell and subcellular organelles, and down to the level of molecular assemblies and single molecules, is important for understanding cellular function. Light microscopy was limited to a resolution of a fraction of a micron by diffraction effects, sufficient for seeing cells and some organelles, but nothing smaller. Later, electron microscopy extended the achievable resolution. Electron microscopy has been extended to higher voltages, allowing thicker, three-dimensional specimens to be examined, including use of 3-D stereoscopic electron microscopy. In addition, entirely new imaging modalities have become available, including acoustic microscopy, atomic force microscopy, and scanning tunneling microscopy. These latter methods allow for imaging structures; contrast is dependent on specimen properties different from those operating in light and electron microscopy. Further, the explosive development of digital methods for image processing has permitted the enhancement of images by means of small, relatively inexpensive computers.

Despite their manifest capabilities, electron micrographic techniques can be applied only to biological specimens that are dead or dying. Obviously this is a serious limitation and has spurred the effort to develop better light microscopic techniques: in the form first of video microscopy and more recently of confocal microscopy.

Confocal microscopes discriminate strongly against information outside the plane of focus. By focusing this plane successively farther into the specimen the microscopes produce an aligned set of 3-D intensity data suitable for analysis and display with the techniques of computer graphics. Although confocal instruments are only beginning to explore the potential of this approach, the 3-D images they produce are dramatic indeed.

Both scanning electron microscopy and confocal light microscopy are sampling techniques, and this simplifies the computer processing of the results. They push older techniques beyond earlier limits and can rapidly produce information-rich 3-D images that accurately represent biological structures on the micro scale.

Light optical microscopy is undergoing a significant expansion of its information-collecting capabilities. Laser sources have made it practical to record diffraction-limited imagery involving gigapixels of digitized information. Confocal scanning microscopes provide optically sectioned imagery of exceptional clarity for thick tissue slices, typically involving data-sets of megapixels. These technological advances have brought about both an increase in data quantity, and the ability to utilize novel, diagnostically useful information. Examples include the detection of changes in the chromatin texture of nuclei, and markers for the presence of malignant lesions of the cervix, thyroid, breast and colon.

The data acquisition capabilities necessitate research into machine vision, and algorithmically controlled image understanding, because image analytic procedures involving extensive human interaction are impractical for data-sets involving the equivalent of thousands of video frames. This in turn raises the question of computer architectures and processing strategies required to extract useful results. Similarly it requires an in-depth analysis of human diagnostic reasoning and the relations between visual diagnostic clues as perceived by the trained human observer and system-computed histometric criteria.

Biotechnology was introduced with a great deal of publicity a little more than a decade ago, and engendered great interest among scientists, as well as among the lay public and investors. It was clear from the beginning that, if the techniques of hybridoma production, monoclonal antibodies, DNA and protein sequencing and synthesis, production of transgenic animals and the like could be well worked out, the consequences for medical diagnosis, therapy, genetic counseling, agriculture and food production would be inestimable. The rush to commercial exploitation may have been somewhat premature, but the variety of procedures for *in vitro* genetic manipulation, in-cell culture and sequencing have been improving steadily. It still remains to be seen how, and in what ways, biotechnology will affect the lives of people, but there can be little doubt of its ultimate practical importance.

For a decade scientists have used monoclonal antibodies as probes to detect the presence of the specific proteins secreted by cells or protruding from the surface of cell membranes. The molecular biologists have shown great ingenuity in tracking down specific macromolecules by this technique. Recently, researchers have begun to attach radioactive labels or pharmacological agents to monoclonal antibodies so that the tagged cells are killed, modified or identified. For example, fluorescent antibodies will permit microscopic identification of tagged cells, or cells tagged with an appropriate chromophore can be irradiated with light (usually by laser) and destroyed. This mode of treatment, called photodynamic therapy, is under active clinical study. In another such study ribosome-inhibiting toxins are being directed in this way to metastatic tumor cells.

Companies specialized in this area are beginning to make a profit. Some are preparing to market cultivated cells and tissues as alternatives to the use of intact animals in toxicity studies. Others have announced their intention to market skin and blood-vessel substitutes that comprise assemblies of cell layers grown in culture to retain desirable properties for grafting, without being rejected by the host.

It may well be that biotechnology offers opportunities for countries to develop uses specific to their needs. Different from the high-technology requirements of many electronic, optical and mechanical devices, biotechnology does not require a large capital outlay at the outset, although it does require a well-trained group of biomedical scientists and technicians, as well as meticulously clean facilities, meticulously maintained, a condition not readily attainable in many countries.

Laser and associated technologies, including electro-optics and fiber optics, are particularly active areas of technology transfer. Some applications, such as laser surgery, are by now fairly common in medical practice. In the United States, 70 % of hospitals with more than 300 beds have at least one surgical laser system. Almost all commercial laser systems being purchased are intended for outpatient surgical procedures. Laser surgery instrumentation is expensive, however: the laser surgery instrument, with the essential peripheral equipment, costs at least $ 100,000.

Laser photodynamic therapy is an area of vigorous research that has shown particular success with bronchial tumors and is being tested against a variety of other types of cancer where the malignant tissue is accessible to an endoscope or an optic fiber and is itself not strongly pigmented: for example, bladder cancer or peritoneal metastases.

Of course, optic fiber technology need not use lasers as its light source. Fiber optic endoscopy has undergone extensive development. The endoscopes can be made quite narrow (1 mm) and possess resolution adequate to permit visualization of blood vessels as small as 3–4 mm in diameter. Already a considerable amount of knee surgery is carried out by arthroscopy, a much less traumatic procedure than the earlier surgical method. The use of light for therapy—an old idea—has been adopted widely by neonatologists for the treatment of jaundice in newborns. Recently, light therapy has been reported to benefit persons suffering from depression. A quite inexpensive portable light source (about $ 150) has been built and tested; it can be worn by the patient (much like a miner's lamp) for several hours, without interfering with customary activities.

A number of companies and academic research groups are exploring the use of laser technology for angioscopy and angioplasty. For example, at the National Institutes of Health (NIH) a team of scientists and engineers has developed an Erbium-YAG laser-based system to open blocked arteries. Laser energy pulses are directed by a special optic fiber against plaque or thrombus. The substances directly in contact with the optic fiber are evaporated to a depth of about one micrometer. The light also induces fluorescence in the fresh surface. The laser firing is controlled automatically by measuring the spectrum of the induced fluorescence of the luminal wall, so that the laser pulse sequence is interrupted once the spectrum is sufficiently similar to the spectrum of normal endothelium. While the procedure has been used successfully on blockages in the superficial femoral artery, the ultimate goal is to ablate plaque in totally occluded arteries, where balloon angioplasty is ineffective. This is a much more difficult task to carry out in tortuous vessels.

Laser technology is also the basis for many measuring devices, especially small, minimally-invasive sensors. Instruments have been developed for transcutaneous, continuous measurement of pH, blood gases, glucose, immunofluorescence, pressure and temperature. Those not commercially available are expected to reach the market in the 1990s. In most instances inexpensive laser diodes may be used as light sources. Nevertheless, currently available measuring instruments are too costly for health care facilities in many developing countries. For example, a laser-based device that entered the market about five years ago to measure blood perfusion in the skin or other accessible tissue surfaces (and which has promise as a diagnostic tool for sickle trait) is commercially available for about $ 10,000.

Another laser-based instrument that may be a candidate for technology transfer assesses the viability of platelets by their optical properties and can evaluate the potential effectiveness of stored platelets, without compromising the sterility of their plastic container. The engineers at NIH who designed and built the device estimate the price of a commercially developed version to be about $ 5,000.

One other research project with great potential application for health in all countries is ultraviolet-light-induced denaturation of DNA in stored blood products. Workers at the Center for Drugs and Biologics, Food and Drug Administration and the Biomedical Engineering and Instrumentation Branch, NIH, have demonstrated the inactivation of a hardy virus (attenuated polio virus) by pulsed ultraviolet radiation at 308 nanometers (an XeCl-Excimer line). Polio virus titers were decreased by 4 to 6 log units, while *in vitro* assays of the irradiated platelets and plasma indicated adequate levels of function. One may anticipate that such studies will ultimately lead to a commercially feasible system for routinely denaturing nucleotide-containing cells, including monocellular or oligocellular parasitic organisms, as well as viruses in blood-bank products.

Within the past two decades, progress in materials science—metallurgy, ceramics, plastics, rubbers, textiles and composites—has had a significant impact on health care. Substances originally intended for non-medical use now play a major role in establishing the quality of performance and longevity of medical and dental devices. Materials can be created to achieve highly specific functions, to fit particular anatomical shapes, and to exhibit predictable properties such as biocompatibility, stability and wear resistance. Many kinds of implant surgery are becoming commonplace. Composite materials are of particular interest because the oriented, woven or lamellar structure of composite materials imparts properties very similar to those of biological composites such as bone, muscle and skin. Composites are being used as internal fracture fixation devices, total joint replacements, ligament and tendon replacements, vascular prostheses and artificial skin. The variety of uses ranges from those required principally for bearing loads to circumstances in which esthetics (for dental surfaces) or complex functional properties (in the case of skin) are paramount.

The technology of drug delivery has undergone extensive development in the last 10 or 15 years. A combination of the disciplines of pharmacology, materials science and device design has brought new concepts to bear in this most ancient therapeutic procedure. The following alternatives to traditional methods of formulating oral medications were listed in a recent publication[2]:

1. Drugs in polymeric capsules in which release is by diffusion through the capsule wall.
2. Drug particles dispersed in a solid matrix with drug release controlled by diffusion through, or erosion of, the matrix.
3. A laminate made by coating a suitable polymer film with solid drug and forming a sealed "sandwich" or "jelly roll".

4. A heterogeneous dispersion of drug in a hydrogel matrix, which controls drug release by slow surface-to-center swelling by water and subsequent drug diffusion from the water-swollen part.

5. Drug encapsulation in a viscous polymer solution.

6. Pumps that either mechanically or chemically (osmotic pressure) deliver the drug at a controlled rate.

7. Drug-coated micropellets with a density lower than gastric juice; the pellets float on the juice while slowly releasing the drug.

8. Drug-containing bioadhesive polymer that adheres to mucin coating the GI tract and is retained on the surface epithelium to extend transit time for the drugs.

9. Chemical bonding of a drug to a polymer backbone by amide or ester linkages, controlling release by hydrolysis.

10. Formation of macromolecular drug composites via ionic or covalent linkages, controlling drug release by hydrolysis, dissociation or microbial degradation.

Analogous principles have been applied to subcutaneous drug implantation. Historically, this was the first medical approach aimed at achieving prolonged and continuous administration. In essence therapeutic devices were prepared by making small, usually cylindrical, pellets. The use of biocompatible polymers to achieve better control of drug release in implantable therapeutic systems followed the accidental discovery of the controlled permeation characteristics of silicone elastomers. Nowadays therapeutic agents can be encapsulated in a variety of ways. The delivery system may be activated by some interaction of the capsule and the body (e.g., osmotic pressure, vapor pressure, temperature, pH) or by external forces (e.g., magnetic, ultrasound, light). Among devices undergoing clinical testing are implanted insulin delivery systems that are activated externally by a digital device, so that the diabetic can administer insulin according to his or her level of activity, type of meal and bodily state.

The third major mode of drug introduction is by intravenous infusion. Recently, it has become evident that the benefits of intravenous drug infusion can be closely duplicated, with fewer of its hazards, by using the skin as the port of continuous drug administration. Several transdermal therapeutic systems have been developed for topical application. They are exemplified by the development and successful marketing of a scopolamine-releasing system (for prophylaxis or treatment of motion-induced nausea), nitroglycerin and isosorbide dinitrate systems for one-a-day medication of angina pectoris, and a clonidine-releasing transdermal system for weekly treatment of hypertension. A number of health care institutions are engaged in developing various transdermal systems for long-term infusion of agents, including antihypertensive, antianginal, antihistamine, anti-inflammatory, analgesic, antiarthritic and contraceptive drugs.

Many other technological areas are being applied to the needs of health care, especially in the industrialized countries. They include such widely accepted procedures as interventional radiology, lithotripsy and heart-assist devices now in use in most urban American general hospitals.

Others are still being tested or are emerging from the research laboratory and beginning to be used clinically. Of particular promise are regional chemotherapy and hyperthermia for adjunctive treatment of localized malignancies, and implanted neural prostheses to provide auditory inputs to patients with severe or total hearing loss and whose cochleas are still intact.

Most of these technologies are costly. The problem for the less developed countries is to determine which are likely to be cost-effective within their economies and appropriate to their level of industrial development. Of course, two-tier medicine is practiced in most countries. Within the upper tier it is very common to find private medicine being practiced with resources fully comparable to those to be found in more affluent countries. Unfortunately, the limited resources of public health-care institutions, whether tertiary or primary, put many of the new devices and systems entirely out of reach.

It is recognized that the first task of a poor country is to develop its human resources. Considerable effort has been extended to training physicians and other health care professionals. However, in my experience, few of these countries or their health ministries have undertaken to train health care professionals in the care and use of modern technology or to create and train the body of technicians required to repair and maintain the new devices.

A few aspects of modern technology can be exploited to the advantage of the poorer countries, if the human resources are available. The prices of virtually every component of modern electronic systems have been lowered so substantially that hardware costs are a small fraction of programming costs. It seems reasonable that "critical masses" of physical scientists, mathematicians and engineers—where they exist—should be motivated to collaborate with health care professionals to develop technologies appropriate to their countries' needs. Many of the devices and systems marketed in the developed countries can be redesigned and built at a small fraction of commercial prices. In following such an approach the principal design criteria need to be simplicity of operation and economics, even if quality must be sacrificed. Cost-effectiveness is perhaps the major criterion. For example, when considering redesign of a CT scanner, one may ask: "How many diagnoses would be missed with a CT scanner that had only half the resolution of the best available ones?" An extracorporeal lithotripter can be designed for local manufacture without a special patient table or X-ray equipment. The cost might be as little as 10% of the current price of about $ 1,000,000. It would entail greater inconvenience for patients and operators, and take more time and perhaps greater skill on the part of the radiologist. Would it be worth it? As with other areas of technological development, it may well be that the best is the enemy of the good.

This synopsis of the current state of affairs in biomedically-oriented technology is put forward by an engineer concerned primarily with research. It may be useful for the purposes of this conference to know the views of the industry. Earlier this year the Health Industry Manufacturers' Association examined "the key technologies and external influences

that will shape the future of the medical device technology industry."
The section of its report dealing with key technologies is appended to this
paper (Annex)[3]. Although the HIMAs' list is derived from the perspective of American industry and describes the state of affairs in industrialized countries, there are some elements that may have relevance for
technology transfer, specifically the emphasis on quality management-
leadership and new manufacturing technologies, two ideas that are
readily appreciated and ought to be readily transferable.

References

[1] Margulis, A.R. The Cutting Edge of Tomography. An abstract for the Drexel
    University-Stein Conference on Imaging in Medicine and Biology: Current
    Issues and Prospects, September 6–8, 1989, Philadelphia, PA.
[2] Hui, Ho-Wah, Robinson, J.R., and Lee, V.H.L. Design and Fabrication of
    Oral Controlled Release Drug Delivery Systems, pp 374–375. In: Controlled
    Drug Delivery: Fundamentals and Applications, Second Edition, Robinson,
    J.R. and Lee, V.H.L. Eds., Marcel Dekker, Inc., New York, 1986.
[3] Willingmyre, G.T. and Estrin, N.F. Strategic Technologies and External
    Influences on the Future of the Medical Device Technology Industry. An
    Executive Summary of a report for the Health Industry Manufacturers
    Association (HIMA), Science and Technology Section, 4 pp, 1989. HIMA–
    1030 15th Street, N.W., Washington, D.C.

ANNEX

Extract of Executive Summary of a report entitled Strategic Technologies and External Influences on the Future of the Medical Device Technology Industry (Science and Technology Section), prepared for the Health Institute Manufacturers Association (HIMA) Washington D.C., U.S.A.

KEY TECHNOLOGIES

While there are undoubtedly many technologies that will shape the future of the medical device and health care industry through the next decade and century, HIMA attempted to identify the few key technologies that are likely to have the most dramatic impact in the next few years and on which HIMA can have impact.

I. New sterilization techniques

The manufacture of sterile device products such as needles, syringes, catheters, and procedure kits depends upon the ability to use effective and efficient sterilization techniques. By definition, sterilization techniques are dangerous processes. They are intended to render products free of microbial contamination. Any procedures with such deadly effects must be carefully controlled and the side-effects of the procedures for the workers, health care professionals and patients considered. At present, techniques for sterilization include: ethylene oxide [EYO] and other chemicals, radiation, heat and steam, and electron beam. For the near future, ethylene oxide represents a very efficient and economical means to render products sterile. If new techiques are to be attractive, they must compete with the efficiency and economics of ETO gas sterilization. However, there is also great potential for new techniques to substitute or replace any of the existing technologies if the substitutes can be safer than present procedures.

II. Quality management leadership

While the industry strives to bring the highest quality products to the U.S. and international marketplace, there are many new quality management concepts that may be brought to bear to maintain this same level of quality at a lower cost or to improve the level of quality. Techniques such as computer-aided design, computer-integrated manufacturing, just-in-time manufacturing, and others need to be brought to bear to assure that the U.S. medical device industry produces the highest quality devices at the least possible cost.

III. Communication and computer technology

The role of micro-processors and software techniques will continue its rapid growth through the next decade and the next century. Software and computer based medical device performance improvements are certain to occur as computer hardware becomes less expensive and software becomes more powerful. Computer information systems will better manage the delivery of health care and networks between and among medical devices, and information systems will be constructed to improve clinical decision-making. Questions of system inter-compatibility and safety must be anticipated and addressed by the industry and future users of computer-based and software-driven instrumentation and information systems.

IV. Date storage and management

The capacity to store and retrieve large bodies of data may change the way in which clinical information is used in the delivery of health care and clinical decision making. Already picture archiving and communications systems (PACs) have the potential to replace silver-based x-ray film. The personal magnetic card medical history has just begun to be used. The paperless medical record is not far behind.

V. Animal substitutes

Today, the use of animal tests for clinical trials of new medical devices is unavoidable. Searches for alternatives to the animal model, however, may pave the way for less use of animals in the future. Scientific breakthroughs in the use of non-living models to evaluate the clinical efficacy and safety of new products will have a major impact in the next century.

VI. New manufacturing technologies

As noted above under "New quality concepts", there are also new manufacturing technologies that can be brought to bear for the medical device industry to produce its products more efficiently. The smaller business community may represent the very best potential for the introduction of new manufacturing techniques to reduce costs and raise efficiencies.

VII. Safety and efficacy testing

Concepts for testing the safety and efficacy of medical devices are presently based upon compliance with standards, test methods and laboratory analyses. There may be new methods for safety and efficacy testing, including alternatives to animal testing, now-destructive techniques such as lasers and holographs, and linking of the results of safety and efficacy testing beyond safety to include relative effectiveness.

VIII. New materials

There is great potential for new materials to be incorporated in medical devices. These include: ceramics, super-conductive products, new sterilizable products, and products that may be acceptable for long-term implants in artificial hearts and orthopedics.

IX. Biosensors

Biosensors will provide the capacity to measure physiological and chemical properties and translate the readings directly to measurable signals. Potential uses include substitution for conventional laboratory tests, and possibilities in biofeedback and closed-loop drug delivery systems.

X. Drug device combination products

More and more frequently the distinction between medical devices and pharmaceuticals is blurring. Devices are becoming intertwined with drugs, as in the case of spermicidal condoms, or the use of contrast agents with imaging techniques, or implantable infusion pumps for drug delivery, or the use of gallstone dissolvers with electro-hydraulic lithotripters. The results of pharmaceutical and device research will bring together new concepts, technologies, and combinations that have not been previously imagined.

ASSESSMENT AND COST-EFFECTIVENESS IN TECHNOLOGY TRANSFER

E.O. Attinger*

Health care has been a preoccupation of mankind throughout history, taking all possible forms between highly individualistic care and socialized systems. Because of resource constraints, compromises between the two extremes have always been necessary. Economics and living standards are powerful mediators for both use and availability of medical technology. Use is also promoted heavily by advertisements of different kinds. Technology more than science moves forward in a world in which time and money have become of prime importance. This leads quite naturally to the temptation to put products on the market without sufficient testing.

However, particularly under conditions of severely constrained resources, the utilitarian doctrine of ethics (the greatest good for the greatest numbers) and the principle of eminent domain in property law (social interests prevail over private interests when they conflict) should become the principal guides for politicians and policymakers, even if they increase opportunity costs in the short run.

Clearly the major health problems of developing countries are different fom those of the developed countries. This paper first describes some of the constraints to the development of health care in developing countries and then discusses some of the features of the most expensive health-care systems in the world, where the results prove once again that money alone is not sufficient to provide health for all the members of a society. This approach has been chosen because much can be learned from the serious mistakes that have been made. A general discussion of medical technology and some of the choices for its application to developing countries constitute the main part of the paper.

More than 80 % of the world's population lives in developing countries and there is every indication that this proportion will continue to grow for the foreseeable future[1]. The growth rate is highest in the poorest countries (2.7%), except for India and China, which firmly enforce population growth programs. Table 1 illustrates some characteristics of the five country groups analyzed by the staff of the World Bank. Although per capita income in the developing countries is still less than 5% of that in the industrial nations, they have shown considerable progress in the statistics for infant mortality, caloric supply and school enrolment. However, infant mortality and life expectancy are still unacceptably high. While the caloric supply would appear adequate in quantity, it is still deficient in quality. Also, these overall statistics

---

* Professor, School of Engineering and Applied Science, University of Virginia, Charlottesville, Virginia, USA.

hide any unequal distribution. Frequently excess consumption by the rich, harvest failures, and spoilage of food in storage and during transport reduce the available supply to starvation levels. Even in the United States more than one seventh of the population has to live below the poverty level[2] while only 4% accounts for nearly half of the national health expenditure. This is, of course, the consequence of a health care system that is highly fragmented and where critical care and life-prolonging procedures are emphasized without regard to societal costs.

In this context, technology has assumed increasing importance, particularly in industrialized countries, where health care expenditures now represent significant fractions of gross national product. In the United States these expenditures have increased more than tenfold over the last two decades, reaching nearly $ 2,000 per capita, or more than three times the average per capita income in the developing countries. Associated with the improvement in the economic status of the population in the industrialized countries, significant changes have occurred in morbidity and mortality patterns. Violence, accidents, drug addiction and chronic diseases such as cardiovascular disease, cancer and metabolic diseases now dominate the scene[3]. At the same time, social institutions as well as families are beginning to disintegrate, indicating a pressing need for more and better education and mental health services. The increase in society's expenditure on medical care may constitute a stabilizing force necessary to counter the destabilizing impulses generated by continued economic development.

It is surprising that in many countries the license to practice medicine still includes unlimited direct or indirect access to the most sophisticated technologies, which require extensive specialized training for their proper use. Indeed, many expensive new technologies, such as magnetic resonance imaging or CAT scans were available in private offices before health care institutions could begin to acquire them. Of course, the astonishing advances in medicine would not have been possible without modern technology, and technology can be expensive[4]. For example, critical care medicine and surgery depend greatly on complex and expensive life-support systems and monitoring equipment but serve only a small fraction of the population. (In 1975 over 50% of spending on acute medical services in the U.S.A. was on behalf of only 4% of the patient population.) This inordinate consumption of resources within one section of society deprives many others of essential requirements such as food and housing.

Many believe that this massive increase in cost has been due largely to excessive use of modern medical technology and have called for a critical assessment of the proper role of technology and its cost-effectiveness in health care. This latter term is often used very loosely[5,6]. By "cost-effective" we mean that a cost-saving procedure can be performed with the same or better result than a more expensive alternative. In cost-benefit analysis, costs are compared with the expected benefit, but the quantification of the latter, in terms of quality life-years gained, for example, is fraught with problems.

Nevertheless, more quantitative methods for analyzing and managing complex systems are essential if we are to make even a beginning in providing health care to all the population. Our obsession with reductionism has led us to ignore the very real values of a systems-oriented approach[7].

Technology has been defined as the body of tools emerging from the interplay of scientific knowledge and practical operation applied to specialized purpose[8]. The term includes medical technology (specialized technology applicable to the practice of medical care, including techniques, drugs, procedures, products and systems combining these elements). Equipment-embodied technology comprises medical technology primarily dependent upon capital equipment to perform health-care tasks, while clinical technology consists of medical technology used in direct patient care. Finally, ancillary technology describes medical technology used directly to support clinical services, such as radiology or clinical laboratories, and coordinative technology represents technology used to facilitate and support the provision of health care services, including administration, transportation and communication, both within and among health-care facilities. Technology assessment is a form of policy research that examines short- and long-range social consequences of the application of technology.

Although in recent years a number of new technologies have been evaluated in a variety of countries, few countries have established mechanisms for systematic evaluation of new medical technologies other than drugs. Such mechanisms are an esential ingredient for establishing and maintaining quality of medical care as well as for the protection of patients and physicians.

Rehabilitation programs constitute an important part of a comprehensive health care system, not only for victims of accidents and trauma, but also for those who suffer from chronic diseases. Particularly for older people with chronic diseases, such services can greatly improve quality of life. Organ transplants of many types are now frequent. Implantable cardiac pacemakers and muscle stimulators are part of the modern medical " tool-box ". Prostheses can permit nearly normal function of the replaced part. However, particularly in this area, successful re-education is a prerequisite for optimal use, and large cadres of professionals are required in this effort—surgeons, immunologists, physicians, psychiatrists, nurses, rehabilitation engineers, occupational therapists, counsellors and a variety of technicians. Also, costs increase disproportionately with increasing levels of complexity in rehabilitation. At the same time, crutches and the more simple prostheses can be produced locally with indigenous materials and enable the patient to achieve a functional level of physical independence for re-integration into society.

In a well-designed system, health-care services should be adjusted and matched to socially and professionally determined health care needs[9]. In practice, however, the needs are often generated either directly or indirectly by the providers themselves for a variety of reasons, including not only humanistic concerns but sometimes also self-interest. In a medical climate increasingly characterized by competition, covert advertisements and public-relation efforts have become accepted practice.

The health problems of the developing countries are still quite different from those of the industrialized West, and call primarily for non-medical measures to improve health: adequate nutrition, sanitation and housing. Although vaccination and immunization have decreased mortality, particularly in infants and children, life expectancy is still unacceptably low. One of the most promising means of raising health levels is a comprehensive effort at general education as a base upon which health-care systems may be built. Transfer of expensive modern technology (technological philanthropy) directed at individual patients would benefit the relatively few rich and leave the remainder in the quagmire of poverty and disease.

A comprehensive prevention program[17] should include four areas in the political-social arena. Prosperity and political action lead to or stimulate better nutrition, housing and the abatement of most environmental hzards. In regard to lifestyle, the need is for interventions successful in unhealthy practices such as smoking and alcohol abuse, sedentary life-styles, accident control and better health practices. In the traditional public health area, health education, immunization, and sanitation must be emphasized. Finally, in the traditional medical care area, a periodic health examination, including preventive measures, can be effective. However, the physician's office is probably the least productive site for prevention. Physician-assistants and nurses are generally better skilled for this type of comprehensive effort. Gori and Richter[18] have estimated that the prevention potential for the five major life-threatening diseases in the USA (cardiovascular, neoplastic and respiratory diseases, accidents and diabetes) ranges from 20 to 80%. As a result of the elimination of these hazards, not only would people profit from a better quality of life, but also their lifespan would be extended considerably beyond the working age.

It is now increasingly realized that medical care represents only a part of a health-care system. Myrdal[10] cautioned against oversimplifying our understanding of health by isolating it from other socioeconomic, institutional and policy aspects of the development process. Stallones also supports this position by the statement that medical care has little, if any, effect on the health of a community, because from a community-health viewpoint medical care always comes too late[11]. However, from a strictly humanistic point of view we must recognize that poor people are willing to use a large part of their resources to alleviate the suffering caused by ill health, though, of course, their sacrifices may be ineffective[12]. The positive impact of comprehensive primary health care has been well documented by Evans[13].

While in industry technology is continuously changing, in the medical sector only relatively few innovations have been applied in practice. Most of the technological changes consist of fancy repackaging. A recent report indicates that the total number of tests and procedures per hospital stay have remained relatively unchanged[14]. However, other authors claim that the use of diagnostic tests and procedures is excessive[15], particularly since most diagnoses can be established with information obtained from a thorough history and physical examination. A case in point is the clinician's ability to estimate the likelihood of coronary artery disease on the basis of sex and the pain pattern in many patients with chest pain. The proper selection and interpretation of diagnostic tests and procedures also require that physicians have easy access to up-to-date, readily retrievable information about them.

The life-cycle of a health technology comprises the stage of emergence, its introduction, adoption and, if necessary, modification in the market-place until it becomes obsolete. For a technology to be successfully transferred, problems and needs must be carefully examined by both the transferer and the transferee. The necessary infrastructure should be available, although modifications may be necessary to meet local needs and resources. Adequate communication and information systems are essential[16].

I have already stated that medical care is not the most important aspect of health care. This becomes apparent when one considers the primary determinants of health: education, communication and trans-portation, adequate housing, nutrition and sanitation. Education for all should emphasize the individual's responsibility for his or her health through health education. Communication and transportation systems as well as coordinating services directed by competent managers are essential for the infrastructure of any society. Adequate housing, nutrition and sanitation must be provided for all, and health services should be coordinated in collaboration with other social services. Smith and Bryant[17] have emphasized the pivotal role of the district for matching local needs and priorities with national policy guidelines and resource allocations. Playing this role effectively requires adequate decentralization of both responsibility and resources. Mechanisms and opportunities for such dialogue already exist within districts in most countries. This model can accommodate the concerns about both accelerating the application of known and effective technologies, and strengthening of community involvement and intersectoral action for health.

References

1. *Social Indicators of Development* 1987. The World Bank, Washington, D.C., 1987.
2. *Money Income and Poverty Status in the USA, 1987.* US Dept. Commerce, Bureau of the Census, Washington, D.C., 1988.
3. *Health United States* 1987, US Dept. HHS, Washington, D.C., 1988.
4. Attinger, E.O., Impacts of the Technological Revolution in Health Care, *IEEE Trans. EME*-31: 12, 1984.
5. Fuchs V.R., What is CBA/CEA and Why Are They Doing This to Us? *New England Journal of Medicine* 303: 937–938, 1980.
6. Doubilet, P., Weinstein M.C. and McNeil B.J., Use and Misuse of the Term "Cost Effective" in Medicine. *New England Journal of Medicine* 314: 253–256, 1986.
7. Christian, B., Kay, D. Benyoussef, A. and Tanashani, T., Health and Socio-economic Development, an Intersectoral Model. *Social Science and Medicine* 11: 63–69, 1977.
8. Medical Technology and the Health Care System. The National Research Council, NAS, Washington, D.C., 1979.

9 Attinger, E.O., *Societal Systems, Technology and Health.* Geneva, World Health Organization 1988.
10 Myrdal, G., *Asian Drama, An Inquiry Into the Poverty of Nations,* Pantheon, New York 1968.
11 Stallones, R.A., Environment, Ecology and Epidemiology. *Who Chronicle* 26: 294, 1972.
12 Candau, M.G., *WHO Chronicle* 25: 441, 1971.
13 Evans, J.R., Hall, K.L. and Warford, J., Health Care in the Developing World. *New England Journal of Medicine* 305: 1117–1127, 1981.
14 Showstack, J.A., Schroeder, S.A. and Matsumoto, M.E., Changes in the Use of Medical Technologies 1972–1977. *New England Journal of Medicine* 306: 706–112, 1982.
15 Griner, P.F. and Glaser, R.J., Misuse of Laboratory Tests and Diagnostic Procedures. *New England Journal of Medicine* 307: 1336–1339, 1982.
16 Panerai, R.B. and Attinger, E.O., *Information-System for Appropriate Allocation of Health Care Technologies,* Medinfo 86, R. Salamon, B. Blum, M. Jorgensen (eds.), Elsevier Science Publ. North Holland 1986.
17 Bonham, G.H., The Four Areas of Prevention Care. *J. Publ. H.* 76: 8–10, 1985.
18 Gori, B. and Richter, R., Macroeconomics of Disease Prevention in the USA. *Science,* 200: 1124–1130, 1978.
19 Smith, D.L. and Bryant, J.H., Building the Infrastructure for Primary Health Care, *Social Science and Medicine* 27: 909, 1988.

ETHICAL ASPECTS OF TECHNOLOGY TRANSFER

A.M. Capron*

In the midst of a technical discussion—on transferring, absorbing, and assessing health technologies across cultures—this paper provides a few thoughts on the ethical aspects of technology transfer. Should we see this as a slighting of ethics? I prefer not to. Instead, I regard it as putting ethics in the middle of health care. It seems fitting to place ethics at the center of our discussion. Indeed, I suspect that even if the topic did not formally appear on the agenda of this conference, many participants would raise questions about the effect that ethics has—or ought to have—on technology transfer. After all, we are not only concerned with technological issues—we are asking the question "whose responsibility?" And this is inherently an ethical question. Certainly some of the most heated issues in the field of technology transfer have been generated by the perception that certain actions or certain kinds of inaction were wrong.

I will begin this morning with a meta-ethical focus, by asking: what ethical norms apply? Then I will look at three categories of ethical issues in technology transfer: first, issues arising from research; second, issues arising from the transfer of particular technologies; and third, those that flow from economic development generally. Finally, I will examine whether technology transfer inevitably entails transplanting certain values that attach to the technologies.

I. Metaethics: whose values should guide conduct?

In the past 20 years in the West, there has been renewed attention to the ethical principles that should guide practice. This examination began, not surprisingly, with the core value that lies at the heart of medical practice—that indeed separates medicine as a profession from mere crafts and trades—namely, the promise that the interests of the patient will be placed above those of the physician or anyone else. Regrettably, this value has not always been given primacy in action. There have been chapters in history—indeed, in our own century—when the sacred trust of the profession has been abused in the service of some other ends— sometimes a noble end, such as the progress of scientific knowledge, but sometimes a base one, such as the dictates of an evil state.

Despite these lapses, the medical profession has shown great loyalty to its promise of fidelity to patients' interests. This principle is usually phrased in terms of beneficence, the obligation to do good, although its

* The Law Center, University of Southern California, Los Angeles, CA 90089–0071, USA.

most famous expression, in the Hippocratic tradition, is the injunction *Primum non nocere,* "Above all, do no harm." This teaching of not causing harm—non-maleficence—was especially appropriate when there was little that physicians could do to cure illness: the best course of action was not to make things worse. With the development of strong and effective remedies, the positive duty of beneficence has become more prominent in the last 50 years, although of late we have come to see that sometimes medicine's great powers to do good can also cause great harm.

As central as this value of beneficence is, not only in the Western tradition but also in Islamic medicine, it has a central problem. When the physician pledges to do good for the patient, the question is: good by whose definition? Who will set the goals and define the values—the physician or the patient?

It is here that the major struggles have occurred in the past 20 years in medical ethics—or as we now say, bioethics, to account for the need to move beyond the conscience of the physician to define what uses should be made of the powers of modern biomedicine. As Dr Gezairy stated to the joint conference of the Islamic Organizations of Medical Sciences and CIOMS in Cairo last year, Islam begins with respect for human dignity: "This entails independent decision-making and continuous protection of such independence." So, too, in the Judaeo-Christian tradition, as it became manifest in the modern world over the past two centuries, the concept of self-determination shone like a beacon. In the past 40 years, that beacon was pointed at medicine, and was developed as the principle of autonomy: that a physician should intervene only after making the patient an informed participant in the process and should always respect the patient's wishes and dignity. Finally, in the ethical traditions of all of our cultures, the principle of fair treatment—and, especially, of treating people equitably, in response to their needs and not their station in life—has been enshrined. I think it is correct to say, however, that the principle of justice was not a central part of *medical* ethics—for the ethics of the individual physician are focused on duties owed to the particular patient being treated. As medicine became a more elaborate enterprise—for example, through human experimentation and through the organization of major hospitals and health systems—the commandment of equitable treatment became inevitable.

I have spent a good deal of time in tracing these three central values—beneficence, autonomy and justice—for several reasons. First, I want to remind ourselves that there is a certain tension amongst them. Most obviously, beneficence can become medical paternalism, which is in conflict with autonomy. Likewise, autonomy can become egoistical self-determination, which is at war with justice. And so forth. If we think of the values of medicine as simple, self-evident or fixed, we make a serious error.

However, I have reviewed these principles for another reason, which is even more central to the task of this meeting. The values emerged from an interaction of physicians with society, but they remain *professional* values related largely to the care of individual patients. Turning to the topic of this conference—the transfer of health-care technologies—physicians may find themselves relating to groups, indeed, to whole populations. What does the concept of beneficence mean in this case? Whose autonomy is controlling, and who determines it?

Moreover, we must recognize that physicians are not the major actors in much transfer of health technology; instead, the power often lies with firms and with governments. Perhaps it would be good if firms and governments agreed to be guided by beneficence, autonomy and justice when dealing with people, both in their own countries and abroad. But I think it is naive to think that the mere presence of the adjective " health " modifying " technology " means that the values of health-care professionals will suddenly govern the actions of self-interested firms and governments. This suggests that our first task is meta-ethical: which values system is operative? After all, at present we are seeing celebrated around the world the value system of the market-place: the triumph of Adam Smith's invisible hand, the principle that in maximizing one's own selfish good one maximizes the collective good. Of course, we know of the costs of such a value system when carried to an extreme. But the major corrective we have for it is governmental, as applied to domestic issues. Once we turn to international issues, the norm of competition again returns, and governments routinely act to promote the self-interest of their countries at the expense of others. Do we presume that countries will apply the principle of justice in dealing with one another? And do we presume that they will apply the principle of autonomy internally—to ensure that decisions are made democratically and with respect for human dignity?

Thus, at the outset we cannot take the " values question " for granted. Instead, we must ask: what values should govern technology firms and governments—and not just physicians—in the transfer of health-care technology?

II. What ethical problems attend the transfer of health technologies?

To have a technology to transfer, there must be research. The first problem here—identifying and prioritizing research objectives—is very much an ethical, rather than solely a technical, issue. It rests on such decisions as: what types of knowledge will be sought? toward ameliorating what diseases? with what speed and intensity? Some people may deny the salience of these questions. They may say that biomedical research is too independent and too serendipitous to be manipulated, as these questions imply. But, while we cannot command science to be ready to answer particular questions, it is certainly possible to prioritize certain areas of research—say, infectious diseases over cancer (even if we later decide that cancer is also in part a disease caused by infection). Likewise, the emphasis in supporting science may be on basic research or on applied research.

In making these decisions, the meta-ethical context arises again. The outcome will be influenced by one's ethical reference point. For example, the norms of profit maximization might guide a vaccine-development company to insist on the monopoly profits that can be attained from a patented biological product. If it does research, therefore, it will want to retain the right to patent. But if the World Health Organization is guided by beneficence, not self-interest, it may insist that it will only support vaccine research when the fruits will be made freely available to all potential manufacturers, without the limitations and profits provided by patent. Once a technology has advanced from the basic and animal laboratories to human testing, we face issues about the involvement of human research subjects in assessing the technology's safety and efficacy. If a technology is developed in country A for use in country B, whose standards of research ethics should be applied? Would it make a difference in the answer one gives whether the technology to be tested will be used primarily in a setting like that in which testing is being proposed (such as a developing country) or it is proposed to test it in one setting (a developing country) and to use it primarily at first in another setting (the developed countries)?

The second general issue under this heading revolves around the product (specific technologies) rather than the process of developing the technologies. During this meeting, I suspect that we shall hear of many examples of particular technologies raising ethical issues. I shall mention only two, which arose during the discussions at the CIOMS Conference on Ethics and Human Values in Family Planning, in Bangkok, to illustrate types of issues.

When, if ever, is it appropriate for a country to limit the transfer to another country of a technology that it finds unacceptable domestically? The clearest answer might be that a country should not transfer to another country a technology that it finds unsafe and will not license for use at home. There may, indeed, be situations in which a product is so faulty that failure to restrict or preclude its transfer would seem immoral.

However, I am concerned lest a too ready answer to this question becomes a firm rule of conduct—that is, if we were to say that a country should never transfer abroad a technology that it will not approve for domestic use. Take this example: in the United States, the drug Depo-Provera is not approved as a long-acting contraceptive by injection. Does this mean that American firms should not be willing or able to sell it in Third-World countries? In those countries, where the risks of pregnancy and childbirth are higher than in the United States and alternative means of contraception are less available or less acceptable, Depo-Provera is an accepted drug. Indeed, experience in the developing world may eventually provide a basis for concluding that this drug is suitable for family planning in the United States in certain populations also characterized by unfavorable risk-benefit ratios with present methods of contraception.

A second question arises: whether it is ever ethical for a country to decline to export a product (even one that may be licensed domestically) because of moral or religious objections. The drug RU–486 illustrates this issue today. Since this drug interferes with the progesterone levels necessary for the continuation of a pregnancy, it is deemed unacceptable by people who oppose abortifacients. For reasons of self-interest, the manufacturer does not want to risk attracting the wrath of these people on all its other pharmaceutical products and hence will not supply the drug. Is this ethical, especially in a developing-country context, where illegal abortion takes many maternal lives? Again, the question is: what norms should apply?

The third set of issues about technology transfer are those that flow from economic development generally. The transfer of health technologies is merely part of a process of economic development, which itself relies on both native and transferred technologies. Historically, development is tied to an increased standard of living, improved health and increased longevity. Some of the effects are general (e.g. less infectious disease as a result of improved sanitation), some relate specifically to medical interventions (e.g. vaccination for childhood diseases), and some flow from improved economic security (e.g. reduction in family size leading to improved maternal and child health). However, economic development can also bring the diseases of industrialization and urbanization, as well as the destruction of the natural environment, the adverse health consequences of which may become apparent only gradually. Also, economic development shifts the need for health care: as the population ages, because of economic development, it will face more chronic illness and more need of health services.

III. Do values inevitably get transferred too?

Technologies are not value-free. A particular technology may take on new, and perhaps unanticipated and even unwanted, characteristics in a new setting. Technology may also carry along values which the population to which it is transferred does not want but cannot avoid. For example, *in vitro* fertilization is associated with particular attitudes toward health, such as that infertility is a disease, not a misfortune or a moral judgment. The technology may thus contradict religious teachings. If infertility comes from pelvic inflammatory disease, which in turn comes from premarital sexual promiscuity, then some people may view it as a divine punishment. Should physicians contradict God's will? *In vitro* fertilization is also linked with a particular attitude toward human beings, which regards human life is something to be manipulated to satisfy certain desires or wants, in this case the desires of an infertile couple to have a biological child. More basically, the whole "high technology" enterprise that is modern medicine in the developed world carries profound value preferences, which determine which populations will be helped, what diseases will be treated, and what forms treatment takes. This is more than an issue of tertiary care over primary care or preventive medicine, although the same phenomenon of pride and glamour that distorts health care priorities in developed countries may come into play in the choices of a developing country about the health-care areas on which it will spend its resources. How many

43

immunizations are not done because scarce resources are expended for a CT-scanner?

The larger issues involve the value (or disvalue) that is associated with the actions of people who are not health professionals (such as clergy and family members), or with the relative preference for length of life over quality of life. Regrettably, much of modern technological medicine is better at extending life than at upholding the humanity of the patient. Of course, for many people, the value of being alive is greater than any other value, but we have to recognize that, inevitably, some technologies may carry certain values with them. The important thing is to be aware of this and, if possible, to weigh the ethical consequences when making the choice.

PROBLEMS AND OPPORTUNITIES IN THE TRANSFER OF KNOWLEDGE

B. McA. Sayers*

Technology transfer has its priorities, like any national endeavour. The factors that influence the priorities of choice are: urgency of need, existence of appropriate technology, willingness of the donor country to transfer—and of the partner country to receive—the technology, and the availability of resources and infrastructure to make the transferred technology viable in the context of the receiving country. The major imponderable here is in the last of these factors: the need for a trained group of scientists and engineers within the country to "absorb" and implement the transferred technology.

There is also another element. Anyone embarking on a new enterprise based on another's experience and "know-how" is, in a sense, an "apprentice". From time to time, diminishingly but inevitably, such a person needs recourse to advice in order to solve fresh problems. For psychological or practical reasons, this may not be a trivial difficulty. In many cases, access to continuing advice will be needed by those in charge of implementing the transferred technology; a methodology to provide this advice must be found which will meet the need without requiring ceaseless contact with the donor agency. A solution may lie in a methodology which is designed into the process of transfer itself—making effective use of developments in information technology. It will be argued that different aspects of information technology can facilitate the transfer of technology, assist the training of specialists in the receiving country so as to establish the important "technological human resource" component of the essential infrastructure, and support the provision of continuing help and advice through the availability of computer-based "expert consultative systems".

It is useful to distinguish between the technology to be transferred and any technology that may be brought to bear on the transfer task itself—in all its ramifications. Technology that might be appropriate to be transferred lies at the high-priority end of a continuum of usable technologies. The distribution of priorities is not the same as the range of technological sophistication; "appropriate technology" is not usually "high technology". Nevertheless, it may be effective, and in all respects beneficial, to use the best possible technology to aid the transfer process. Some of the most advanced aspects of information technology, as will be seen, may be highly appropriate in transferring intermediate-level technology to the least developed of countries.

* Professor, Centre for Cognitive Systems, Imperial College of Science Technology and Medicine, London, SW7 2AZ, UK.

The task of setting priorities for technology to be transferred is complex; a need undoubtedly exists for a basis on which priorities can be allocated—preferably an objective basis. Transfer of technology implies the use of resources: of manpower, physical facilities and money. The resources must, very often, be obtained by diversion from other activities or other sectors of the economy. So it is unwise to consider the desirability, regardless of priority, of transferring a given technology, without looking at the same time at the problem which is to be solved by the technology, and at the whole socio-economic context in which the diversion of resources will occur. The full methodology for setting priorities in this way would itself be a widely-transferrable technology; unhappily, it does not yet exist. In the meantime, selecting priorities may be largely a political issue, informed by whatever technical advice and support can currently be provided. Trained personnel are again the key to providing this advice: on the basis of an objective examination of the issue of resource allocation, using the skills of modern computer system analysis and optimisation procedures where these are needed.

To consider the issues of problems and opportunities systematically, one must identify the relevant requirements for successful transfer of technology, and consider what difficulties might inhibit the process, and what problems might imperil the successful implementation of the transferred technology. These matters are interlinked. The perceptions of individuals in the developing country of what technology transfer involves, and what it is intended to achieve, are important; but expectations about the practicalities are equally relevant. Expectations about how the implementation is to be achieved in the country, and about what understanding and insight are necessary, must be realistic. They involve, first, the existence of a "critical mass" of professionals so as to create the appropriate technological environment, and second, the existence of specific capabilities amongst these professionals. A critical mass of professionals is essential to provide the mutual support, and challenge, that maintains standards and offers encouragement to improved efforts; their essential capabilities must include an informed understanding of the basic science underlying the technology (vital to allow design developments to meet the country's specific needs), as well as, of course, the ability to modify fabrication technology to suit the techniques, skills and raw materials available in the country. Without these two prerequisites, successful technology transfer is uncertain.

The need for an appropriate professional infrastructure

Technology never stands still. It never produces the ideal product: always there are improvements to be made, often the need for correction or modification ("fixes"), sometimes compensatory procedures or products to be devised, and consumers—who constitute the market—develop preferences. (Introduction of a new model of motor-car is almost invariably followed by a series of abrupt modifications, sometimes

46

requiring recall of vehicles already on the roads. Use suggests improvements, and features found to be strongly desirable influence subsequent market demand. The introduction of lead and other additives in motor fuel undoubtedly improved engine performance, but now needs a panoply of design changes and devices to prevent or trap unwanted by-products of internal combustion.) So if technology is to be transferred, with the aim of creating an indigenous industry, that industry must have scientists and engineers capable of carrying through all the steps that are vital to establish and maintain a viable industry: devising products, product design, fabrication process design, production and production management, quality assurance, setting up maintenance protocols and procedures, product sales and performance analysis, and supervising trainees. Also, a proportion of them need to be able to work with accountants, economists and managers. In short, transfer of technology demands well-trained—and appropriately trained—technological personnel, with a wide range of skills superimposed on a sound understanding of the scientific bases of the technology.

One of the responsibilities of these professionals is to set up an organization, and train personnel, to provide after-sales service or, in the case of laboratory or non-production technology, maintenance. Product design, whether it involves, say, prostheses or other manufactured artefacts such as medical instruments or equipment, needs to take account not only of the constraints due to the production process but also of the fact that maintenance must be as simple as possible. So the other personnel "arm" of the infrastructure is technician support for maintenance and repair.

Educational requirements

Some of the more persistent problems in successfully transferring technology stem from a lack of perception in the receiving country about the nature of understanding and insight in technology, which is of course, applied science, and about the extent to which scientific understanding is critical, in order to cope with and benefit properly from technology transfer. If the educational traditions are not appropriate, then the manpower infrastructure for technology transfer will not be appropriate. This is partly a matter of practices in secondary and tertiary education.

An unsuitable education probably does not affect the very brightest, who have their own spontaneity of understanding; but it puts at risk the bulk of those who will constitute the country's future professionals. I have had experience with very many senior professional staff from developing countries who have proved, in the outcome, to be both impressive and original—but whose background training suffered greatly from an inability to reason from first principles about problems. This sometimes stems from practices that are unavoidable when an educational system is obliged to cope with large numbers of pupils despite an

47

inadequate numbers of teachers. Necessarily perhaps, it places much emphasis on working through textbook material rather than linking principles and concepts to practical laboratory or workshop studies—an approach that fails to encourage the habits of enquiry and challenge, or of searching for a synthesis of complex arrays of information.

It can certainly be argued, from experience, that the education of scientists and technologists is greatly influenced by traditions in schools, especially secondary schools and universities. The mental habit of enquiring and challenging is important to scientific development but it does not often occur spontaneously, particularly as a well-formed ability: it needs to be recognized, nurtured and encouraged. If this does not happen at school then it must happen at university, or the production of scientifically sound manpower will certainly be compromised.

In terms of technological education, the natural skill that must be recognized and developed is that of synthesis and design. Uninformed individuals sometimes marvel uncritically at the skills of someone who can assemble a useful artefact from highly unlikely and seemingly unsuitable components; but the skill that they should be admiring is the spontaneous gift of synthesis—and the visualisation in the mind's eye of a finished design towards which the assembly grows, element by element. Again, if these abilities are not nurtured and strengthened at school, then it must happen at university—where the "formation" process of the engineer must also include experience of the design process at its most general.

It might be thought that the education of the kind of engineer needed to cope with the transfer of advanced technology is easily specified: ensure that he is equipped by being trained up to the best practice in the latest relevant techniques, so that he leaves his studies fully able to practise immediately as, say, a production engineer or some other technological specialist. However, it is almost impossible to do a thorough job of teaching students in this way if, at the same time, one wishes to ensure that students graduate with adequate ability to follow advances in their professional field. It is salutary to remember that over the last 40 years the specialty of electronic engineering has had to weather five major changes: from thermionic valve technology to transistor technology to integrated circuit technology to hybrid software/microchip technology and finally very large-scale integrated circuits: first digital, then analogue: designed with computer tools. Many electronic engineers who were highly competent in their subject as it was practised when they started in employment were never able to upgrade their understanding to operate effectively in newer technical aspects. The reason was that, despite their efficiency in the technology in which they had been brought up, their basic scientific understanding was not sufficiently sound. This illustrates how essential it is to have a good understanding, especially of physical science (including, of course, chemistry and biochemistry in certain specialties).

What if the developing country does not have a sufficient group of suitably trained professionals to cope with the transferred technology; what can be done to help? The key decision is that the senior engineers who are to take charge of the project must be adequately equipped. However, training senior professionals—especially in basic ways of approach—is not easy, for either tutors or students. Fortunately, experience in handling this task has been obtained in recent years, and there are now satisfactory ways of retraining experienced, senior personnel. These ways use the important pedagogical principle of structuring the retraining programme in the light of the knowledge that these personnel are likely to be highly experienced in practical problem-solving. A computer-based tutoring system can be constructed on this basis, using recent advances from research in information technology—and specifically artificial intelligence.

The matter of teaching specific skills is, at first sight, rather different but here the same recent advances in information technology should certainly be able to help. Techniques of computer-aided learning have advanced very rapidly in the last two years and the new methods will undoubtedly dominate very soon. These make use of aspects of artificial intelligence in order to control the "teaching" process. The student is presented with material stored on a digital video compact disc, using a personal computer display. The controlling system "constructs" an up-dated "model", the controlling system charts a "pathway" through the material to be learned, using archive and text-book material, explanatory text and video, problem questions and other devices as appropriate. In this way, the student's grasp of all relevant background is built up and strengthened, and he is given experience both in using the material and in realistic problem-solving. The "learning strategy" can be tailored to the kind of experience brought by the student to the retraining task.

Naturally, this is only possible when expert knowledge is available of all aspects of the material to be "taught"—that is, the actual "technology" to be transferred. It required the availability of experts in the donor country to allow the educational material to be assembled in such a way that the essential fundamentals and the key techniques are identified, the important areas for practice selected, and the best problem-solving experience decided, from which the right presentations can be planned and the linkage between student "model" and consequential "pathway" can be chosen. It is evident that this approach is no substitute for real experience, in the donor country, of the technology to be transferred. Nevertheless, it does offer the opportunity for preliminary training and follow-up consolidation for the most senior staff, and as the main vehicle for the training of support technologists.

The transfer process

Various factors influence how best to transfer technology. But, as argued above, technological practice cannot safely be transferred without an understanding of the fundamentals, i.e., without the relevant science. So transfer must involve senior, adequately trained scientists and engineers with the appropriate skills.

It is taken as self-evident that the process of transfer will normally involve a period of on-site training of the responsible personnel from the receiving country, in an institution or industry within the donor country. However, particularly if the donor source is industrial, the scientists and engineers of a donor organization are not necessarily teachers. Explaining the science and the technology may not be easy in that case. The process of conveying the essential knowledge, and communicating the best practical procedures and techniques, could be greatly aided by the computer-aided learning techniques mentioned above, although the effort and cost of preparing the tutoring material would need careful justification unless a very substantial group were to be trained. The preparation of tutoring material is, in any case, a specialist task, best carried out under contract by a specialist organization. Once developed, the framework of computer software (but not, of course, the specific detail) can be used again in various different technology-transfer situations.

Another useful resource may also be derived from another aspect of information technology, namely the "expert consultative system". Here again, a knowledge base is formed in a computer, consisting of as much relevant knowledge as can be obtained about the technology to be transferred, including its implementation. Some of this "knowledge" will comprise the basic science involved, some the technological development of the basic idea, some the practicalities of implementation, some the features of good design for that technology, and some the details of "troubleshooting" on the factory floor. Most of it will include both factual information and practical, empirical "rules of thumb" and observations about the "behaviour" of technology, which constitute much of the valuable capability of experts, acquired through years of experience. It is organized, by use of suitable software, in a manner that allows the logical inter-relationships between the various "pieces" of "knowledge" to be identified, and general inferences made. This technology depends upon two recent developments: in the computer representation of "knowledge"—how to record facts, observations and experiential beliefs in the form of verbalized statements with grammatical structure and meaning, not merely as "strings" of characters, in the computer— and in understanding how to use a computer to undertake logical manipulations upon these pieces of "knowledge".

Structured information in a knowledge base would provide implicit expert know-how on solving problems that arise—whether problems of understanding about the technology, or problems in design, production or use. The knowledge base can be interrogated about these matters, and caused to make recommendations about possible courses of action, together with "explanations" of its "reasoning". So, certainly in principle and already to an appreciable extent in practice, the system can be used as an "expert advisor" on the transferred technology to the technologists in the receiving country. It will be seen that, as the science of machine logic improves, this kind of approach is likely to offer precisely the facility needed to optimise the transfer of technology and its use in the receiving country.

Concluding note

The imperatives of successful technology transfer start with urgency of need and finish with the capability to operate and use the technology satisfactorily in the receiving country. The role of the trained personnel who are to receive the technology is vital. They must be sufficiently numerous to constitute a "critical mass", and have the scientific insight and understanding to make full and informed use of the technology—a requirement which has been emphasised throughout the above commentary, and which generates special problems in achievement. However, recent experience should be helpful.

The process of transfer itself can rarely be achieved by the transmission of documents alone. Professionals to receive and operate the transferred technology will often need a period of instruction in the fundamentals involved, practical experience with the technology in the donor organisation, and a period working under supervision. The resources of information technology should be valuable in offering the opportunity to set up not only advanced training procedures, but also an "expert consultative system" in each case, with which the responsible professionals could access "automatic" advice on the solution of problems during implementation. The former would help solve the problem of achieving a satisfactory infrastructure of technical support; the latter would be critical in efficiently ensuring the smooth continuing implementation of the transferred technology.

PROBLEMS AND OPPORTUNITIES IN THE ABSORPTION OF TECHNOLOGY

B.O. Osuntokun

The utilization of well-tried technologies for health care delivery in the developing countries should be considered a top priority. However, developing countries also need to consider the use of the newer technologies resulting from recent advances in biological and physical sciences. These include new approaches to vaccine and drug development, improved diagnostic techniques, early detection of hereditary disorders, the enormous potential for health-care technology of results of biotechnology research, microelectronics and information technology, materials technology and biocompatible materials, systems technology and modelling. Some of the problems and opportunities in the absorption of technology are also common to those encountered in transfer of technology from the "seller" to the "user"—already covered by Professor Sayers. Some of the most important issues in the absorption of technology in developing countries can be summarized as follows:

1. National policy on health-care technology

Most developing countries have no national policy on health care technology. To facilitate health care technology transfer every developing country should have a mechanism to enable it to decide what technologies it needs, for what purpose and at what level of health care. Such technologies must be related to health-care priorities within the context of a national health policy (and national health-related research policy) and should be reviewed from time to time. It is important that such technologies considered as top priorities should be appropriate (see section on Partners in Technology Transfer) and, if possible, with already proved effectiveness and safety, and they must be ethically, socially and culturally acceptable and affordable in terms of cost-benefit and cost-effectiveness. The need for a national policy on health care technology as a prerequisite for transfer and absorption of technology is further discussed in the section on Partners in Technology Transfer. The evolution of a national policy on health technology should involve policy-makers as well as scientists, technologists and health-care practitioners.

---

* Professor, University of Ibadan, Ibadan, Nigeria.

2. Presence of appropriate receptor mechanism for transfer and absorption of technology

Most developing countries have no mechanism to serve as "receptor" for technology absorption. Technology can be absorbed only if the essential components of an effective receptor mechanism are present. These involve (a) a body or "critical mass" of trained personnel with the basic knowledge, skill and capability to harness and maintain the technologies to benefit health care systems; (b) an adequate infrastructure of social services (water, power supply, transport, etc.) and other relevant environmental factors. An attractive career structure is essential if trained personnel are to be retained and brain drain avoided. Training of personnel may be "mission-oriented" or "goal directed" to achieve absorption of specific technology, e.g., training of staff in special institutions and universities in such fields as biotechnology, vaccine production, drugs manufacture, hospital equipment engineering, and medical (intensive) care technology. Local training of personnel on the job would be ideal, but may be inadequate. Training of personnel abroad may involve the risk that some may not return. Training and retraining may need to be intensified if users are to keep up with advances in knowledge. Cost of training especially outside users' countries could be prohibitive because of the foreign exchange component unless it is absorbed by the "seller".

Every effort must be made to ensure adequate maintenance of equipment and of a sufficient stock of spare parts so that the equipment functions. The possibility of local manufacture of equipment or spare parts must be explored.

3. Adequate information system

Few developing countries have a suitable information system for technology. An efficient information system is essential for effective planning of transfer and absorption of technology, for its maintenance and for awareness of the choice of technologies that are needed and are transferable. It also augments training facilities. Every effort must be made to overcome the possible reluctance of "sellers" to make available to the "users" complete information on technology, in order to ensure continuing access of the sellers to the users' market.

4. Research and development

Most developing countries do not have research and development units or their equivalents for technology. Once a country accepts the need for technology transfer and absorption, it must accept that research and development are essential as well. Research and development units must be set up, and may include, where necessary and feasible, consultants from outside the country. Such units would be well placed to advise the country on the choice of technologies to be transferred, absorbed and developed in relation to the country's needs, and could serve as bridges between the user-countries and the "sellers" or suppliers. They would also foster the development of indigenous technologies as well as monitor new and emerging technologies on a continuing basis.

A turn-key approach to technology transfer, i.e. the supply of equipment ready for operation, should rarely be encouraged.

Developing countries must be prepared to invest in research and development based either on technology transfer or on ideas developed from transferred technology or on original ideas. Research and development must include evaluation of absorbed technology for cost-benefit, cost-effectiveness, quality control, and abuse. The essence must always be upheld that the ideal technologies to be transferred to and absorbed by the developing countries are those that assure the greatest benefit for the most people.

As far as possible, research and development units should be based in universities or research institutes, but with representation of the ministries of education, health, science and technology and agriculture, as well as of the community.

6. Deliberate cultivation of a technology science culture

Few of the developing countries have adequate levels of science education. A culture of respect for, and use of, science and technology takes some time to be developed in any community and needs to be deliberately fostered. It may require continuous scientific education of one or two generations before the use of the application of science is accepted for solving problems. It is obvious that certain levels of technology may therefore not be transferable until science education and literacy reach a certain level or until a "critical mass" of trained personnel becomes available.

ROLE OF REGULATORY AUTHORITIES IN TECHNOLOGY TRANSFER

J.C. Villforth*

Importance of communication

The complex role of medical-device regulatory authorities in protecting the public health is magnified many times over when applied to the transfer of health technology. Although we need to take a global view in assessing and addressing public health, we must also be aware of the problems and perspectives of each country. We sometimes tend to oversimplify a situation by placing ourselves into a pigeon-hole of being either a developed or a developing country. Within both there are degrees of difference that merit our attention. Only by communicating the needs of one with the constraints of the other will we begin to understand the tremendous challenge that awaits regulators of medical devices in assuring that technology transfer is safe, effective and appropriately applied.

Developing countries face very serious issues, such as climatic conditions, purchasing specifications, language problems, and training. Considerable resources are required even to transport and get spare parts into countries remote from the place where equipment is manufactured. One of the biggest obstacles to technology transfer is the dearth of trained and qualified people to do the job.

Even the industrialized countries are not uniformly and monolithically developed. There are probably more areas being developed than already developed. One does not have to wander far from the large teaching university hospitals in the metropolitan area of Washington, D.C. to find in our Appalachian region certain medical practices that are not up to the standards of a developed country. Extreme climatic conditions and problems of maintenance and training also exist in so-called developed countries.

It is very important for each of us to convey and appreciate the perspectives of the other. The whole essence of information exchange, and the question of the role of each member nation, the role of each collective organization, and the role of each regional or multinational agreement, depend on how well we can communicate with, and understand, one another. One of the obvious constraints in the transfer of technology is lack of resources.

Limited resources

The resources available for the management of medical devices are limited when we consider the priorities that face public health officials

* Professor, Center for Devices and Radiological Health, Food and Drug Administration, Bethesda, Maryland, USA.

around the world. Problems need to be examined very carefully to ensure that the priorities established focus our attention and apply our resources where the greatest public health need is found. We shall have to work even harder in the future to ensure that critical medical devices are safe and effective. Some of the less risky devices may reach the marketplace without the full degree of scrutiny usually given to the more complex devices.

The world of medical devices

The medical-device industry is extremely diverse. The world of devices ranges from the most complex diagnostic and therapeutic apparatus, involving sophisticated high technology, complex electronics, computer technology, exotic chemistry and materials, to the simplest mechanical devices and laboratory and diagnostic apparatus. *In vitro* diagnostics are of particular interest as medical devices. They are undergoing rapid development and are commonly used by consumers in their homes. Electronics, microprocessors, computers and software complicate the picture, with issues ranging from reliability, safety and effectiveness to the fundamental definition of a medical device.

The disciplines involved in the field of medical devices include medicine, biology, epidemiology, computer science, and all the elements of physics and engineering, as well as such hybrid fields as biomaterials science, biotoxicology, biotechnology and biocompatibility. Ceramics are becoming popular and find increasing use in medical devices. We are increasingly concerned with the effect of bioenvironments on the strength of metals and other materials, on ceramics, and on polymers. All of these complications demand a high degree of sophistication and scientific competence on the part of the public health regulator.

New technology

Another complexity of medical devices is related to their accelerating rate of technological development and technology diffusion. This places a very heavy burden on regulatory authorities struggling to keep abreast of developments in medical-device technology. Only a few years ago the cochlear implant was approved in the United States. It is now having a big impact on those who are totally deaf, providing a sensation that assists them in lip-reading. Intraocular lenses have been in use for some time and are increasingly accepted. The neodynium-YAG laser has replaced conventional surgery for lens replacement capsulotomy. Newer technologies involving the excimer laser are on the horizon, providing an additional mechanism of photochemical action for use in delicate surgery on the eye and other tissues.

Fiber optics as a means of visualizing internal body structures and collecting important diagnostic information may affect future *in vitro* diagnostic product technologies. Artificial intelligence will help the clinician in the diagnosis of disease and the determination of the course of the patient's well-being. The complexity and rapidly changing field of medical devices will provide increased pressure on public health officials to stay on top of the technology and to make maximum use of their limited resources.

May devices are now being introduced in combination with drugs. Some examples are: the heparin and antibiotic-coated catheter, intended to prevent clogging formation and to enhance the device's performance; and the steroid-tipped pacemaker lead, intended to avoid inflammation of surrounding tissue. Work is being done on how best to "manage" the regulation of these devices in order to avoid dual requirements by both the drug laws and the device laws. Manufacturers in the U.S.A. will need to inform the Food and Drug Administration (FDA) early when a device is being developed so that a decision can be made on how it should be regulated. At the same time, the FDA will need to provide more guidance to manufacturers of innovative products.

Regulation of medical devices

As the device industry evolves, so does the regulation of medical devices. Countries have diverse approaches to regulating medical devices. Programs range from no regulation at all, to the stringent system of regulation of the U.S.A., to the British system, which uses the "purchasing power" of a device to determine whether it will be marketed. There is a need for countries to establish local regulation of medical devices and to clearly identify their requirements so that any new programs established in the international arena can be integrated into a country's existing program. Even though there is no master plan or universal means for regulating medical devices, a common framework can be established by using those principles found in existing regulatory programs.

The regulation of medical devices began in the U.S.A. with the 1976 Medical Device Amendments to the Food, Drug, and Cosmetics Act. The Amendments gave the Food and Drug Administration authority to ensure that medical devices marketed in the U.S. are safe and effective for their intended use. The level of control applied to a device is based on its level of risk to health. The principal burden of proving safety and effectiveness lies with the sponsor, usually the manufacturer. External reviewers, such as peer review groups or advisory panels, examine the data and make recommendations for action. We believe that the U.S. regulatory controls are strict enough to be a challenge and yet not so strict as to inhibit innovation.

Decisions to approve a device for marketing are based on scientific data that must show both safety and effectiveness of the device's intended or labelled use. A device's cost-effectiveness is not considered during this approval process, although the information gleaned from clinical trials on safety and effectiveness can be applied by insurers who do cost-benefit analyses to establish reimbursement fees for devices and clinical procedures.

Classification of devices

Because of the large number of medical devices (about 1700 generic types) and the wide variation of risks among them, the Amendments establish a three-tiered system of regulatory classification—Class I, Class II and Class III—based on device risk. Both new devices and those found to be substantially equivalent to already marketed devices are placed into one of these three classes.

Pre-market approval

Device manufacturers must notify FDA in advance of their intent to market a device. The law gives FDA the authority to call for additional clinical data in those cases where changes to the device's intended use or a change in its design, material, chemical composition, energy source or manufacturing process could affect its safety or effectiveness.

The uterine monitor, on the market prior to the 1976 amendments, is used in hospitals and other clinical settings to detect uterine contractions to determine preterm delivery. When manufacturers applied to FDA to market the device for home monitoring, a use that goes beyond its intended use, FDA required that clinical studies be conducted and scientific data be submitted to substantiate claims of safety and effectiveness for this new use. Another example is the Doppler ultrasound device, already on the market to detect heart rate in adults and children. Additional clinical data were called for when manufacturers decided to market the device to detect the fetal heart rate.

Registration, listing, labeling and Good Manufacturing Practices

Under the amendments, manufacturers must also register their establishments with FDA, list their products, comply with labeling requirements, and follow Good Manufacturing Practices (GMP). FDA field inspectors periodically inspect manufacturing facilities to assure compliance with GMP. The law allows for product recalls and follow-up inspections of facilities not in compliance.

Performance standards

Another provision of the Medical Device Amendments requires that performance standards be established for products falling into certain categories. Although few mandatory performance standards have been set, much work has been done with the voluntary-standards community in establishing and maintaining voluntary performance-standards. The FDA Center for Devices and Radiological Health (CDRH) has participated in more than 200 standard-setting functions, both domestic and international.

While most of the efforts in voluntary standards development have been in device-specific or so called "vertical" areas, the Center is particularly interested in the development of generic, or horizontal, standards. The current horizontal standards approach of the European Community (EC) is one that CDRA favors. As a first priority, EC standard-setting activities will be directed toward the development of horizontal standards for good manufacturing practice, biocompatibility, labeling and sterility. We feel that the establishment of horizontal standards is an efficient, a cost-saving, and an effective way to address many public health concerns.

The world is moving more to international standards as the medical-device community becomes more interdependent. There is a need to form stronger international organizations where public health authorities cooperate in setting standards so that more public health concerns are considered when standards are being written. International standards will be helpful in assuring consistency and in protecting product liability. We support and encourage increased communication and collaboration with our colleagues around the world to work toward harmonization of medical-device standards. However, we are aware that, even after international standards are set, the difficult task of implementation will remain.

Reporting

As part of our regulatory efforts, CDRH maintains data-bases that require device manufacturers to report to FDA any deaths and serious injuries related to medical-device use, and device malfunctions that could cause death or serious injury. Unfortunately, the value of this information is limited unless it can be communicated to every country where the device is being sold.

How do we communicate data on adverse reactions or recalls to every country that would benefit from this information? Currently, the United States goes through the State Department. However, we cannot be assured that the information gets into the hands of health professionals in hospitals and other clinical facilities, or to suppliers, distributors or consumers. Our recall data go into the Emergency Care Research Institute (ECRI), and Canada is using our data-base, and we shall be using theirs. But it is important that all nations have the ability to share device data in a common data-base.

Research on medical devices

Research data-bases are also needed. CDRH considers it essential to maintain an active research base, even during these times of limited resources. We believe the existence of a research science base permits us to make the best use of available information, and to generate new information at times, both of which help us to feel more assured about our public health decisions and our evaluations of problem products. Generally speaking, CDRH medical-device laboratories provide crucial support and input for the Center's product approval, postmarketing surveillance and user education programs. They also provide the Center with an independent means for addressing fundamental public health issues, both in forecasting upcoming problems and in developing technological improvements or "fixes" that may help to solve key problems.

The laboratory program includes a mix of both forward-looking developmental projects and work of immediate applicability on problems facing us now. This includes the analysis of phenomena that cut across broad device-areas, such as understanding the properties of the various types of materials used in devices, and problems of equipment automation.

We believe our research efforts are enhanced through collaboration with other scientific groups outside the Center, both in the U.S. and in countries around the world. Scientist-to-scientist collaboration has allowed CDRH to multiply its resources substantially in many areas. Within the U.S., CDRH maintains cooperative efforts not only with the other parts of the Food and Drug Administration, but also with the National Institutes of Health, the National Bureau of Standards, the Occupational Safety and Health Administration, and the National Aeronautics and Space Administration (among others). Research collaboration and measurement intercomparisons involve many countries in the Western hemisphere and Europe, as well as Australia, Japan and the Soviet Union. This effort includes not only continual inter-laboratory contact and collaboration but also a visiting-scientist program in which senior professionals spend extended periods working on projects of joint interest in the Center's laboratories. In addition to such governmental collaboration, CDRH collaborates extensively with university and other research groups. To help identify and establish our global research priorities, all countries will need to make known their health needs and to share their existing research data.

The field of medical devices is so broad that CDRH must focus its developmental work. CDRH undertakes four categories of work: first, things others cannot do, perhaps for lack of expertise or equipment; second, things others will not do, for lack of adequate incentive, financial or other; third, things others should not do, such as maintaining the only source of information on product failures; and finally, things others have not done, to fill gaps in our knowledge.

FDA is currently doing research on the DNA hybridization probe as part of a continuing effort to build up in-house expertise that can be applied to the Agency's review process. New *in vitro* diagnostic products are likely to be generated by this initiative. A major thrust has begun with the development of a DNA probe that will be used to detect arenavirus, which causes hemorrhagic fever in a significant portion of the population in South America, Asia and Africa. The U.S. is the only part of the world where strains of arenavirus causing hemorrhagic fever are not found. This project will have practical application to the military and to

Third World countries, but it is an area of research unlikely to be developed by U.S. industry.

Sharing research on particular device problems would also benefit countries. Additional epidemiological data would help to determine how to detect potential device problems before they occur. The U.S., the United Kingdom, and Canada are interested in sharing epidemiological data on heart-valve failures so that potential failures can be detected before they occur. Heart valves are worn by 60,000 people around the world. Some researchers are questioning the possible effect that a collagen implant has had on autoimmune disease. As a result of this, FDA has renewed its interest in looking at results of scientific studies on the collagen implant. A reliable research base provides benefits not available from any other source.

Educational activity

We have found that the education and training of users of medical devices also provide benefits. Apart from the problems of the mechanical failure of a device *per se*, there are failures that may be the result of user error. Whether the user be the clinician, the technologist or the consumer, we must develop educational programs to inform and educate the professional user and the public about potential problems in order to avoid them and to improve the use of the device. We must work with the clinicians, the consumers, and the technologists to bring this about. We realize that we cannot do it at the Federal level by ourselves: we must start to develop ideas and concepts that can be multiplied and expanded by professional organizations, consumer groups, and international organizations to extend the limited resources that we have available to get the job done. The multiplier effect will supplement our resources and amplify our activities in the U.S. and, we hope, throughout the world.

By increasing our awareness of global problems through conferences such as this, regulators of medical devices can begin to work together toward funding and implementing solutions that will satisfy, at the very least, our most critical needs.

PARTNERS IN TECHNOLOGY TRANSFER

Perspectives of Industrialized and Developing Countries

TECHNICAL COOPERATION AGENCIES AND HEALTH TECHNOLOGY TRANSFER

Rolf Korte*

Objectives and principles of technical cooperation

The objective of technical cooperation is the well-being of broad population groups in developing countries. It is achieved by the transfer of both know-how and materials, by means of consultants, materials and finance, and by education and training. A guiding principle is to act only at the request of recipient governments and to involve target groups as early as possible in the formulation and implementation of projects and programmes. The technologies must be appropriate in the development context.

It is a characteristic of German technical cooperation that no funds are specifically earmarked for the health sector: health has to compete with other activities for funding. Therefore the level of funding reflects the generally low priority afforded to the health sector, as evidenced by the reduced allocations to health budgets, which have shrunk by 50 % during the last 10 years in proportion to total government spending.

While German technical cooperation programmes are only rarely obliged to supply specific brands, this is not the case with many donors, regrettably. Yet, product choice, even in the absence of restrictive regulations, is frequently determined by the familiarity of donors with their own markets.

This paper discusses technology transfer as observed in the context of German technical cooperation. The objectives and principles of other donor countries may differ, but most problems in technology transfer are common to all partners, regardless of their implementation mechanisms.

Technology is a broad term which is used to denote the technical tools required for diagnosis, treatment and prevention, as well as know-how in general, including aspects of training, management and organization. This paper considers only technical tools, but includes a brief discussion of some aspects of drugs, immunology, genetics and information science, which are often not counted as tools.

Also the term "developing country" requires some definition, as the level of development and therefore technological appropriateness varies significantly between developing countries. For example, a magnetic resonance imaging system may be justifiable for China but not for one of the least or less developed countries.

---

* Health, Population and Nutrition Division, Deutsche Gesellschaft für Technische Zusammenarbeit (GTZ), GmbH, Eschborn, Federal Republic of Germany.

Priority programmes and activities of the German Association for Technical Collaboration (GTZ)

In the health sector German technical cooperation activities follow the guiding principles elaborated by the World Health Organization. Primary health care programmes therefore form the largest part of project activities. More recently the provision of primary health care within district health services has been re-emphasized. With the present economic crisis, especially in Africa, technical assistance in this field has become extremely difficult. Even the most modest inputs are in danger of not being sustainable. In many countries that show the availability for health-care services of US $ 5 per caput a year the figure is misleading as it does not reflect the uneven distribution of resources within the countries; for many rural populations the amount may be closer to US $ 1–2.

Family planning is a major concern of our work in the health sector, because of the widespread scepticism within industrialized countries about the advisability of getting involved in this area, while the demand remains high. We know that the technologies available are not ideal, but when a risk evaluation is made all methods, except unsafe abortions, are less risk-laden than unwanted pregnancies.

The control of infectious diseases, including immunization, has normally been effected by vertical programmes. Attempts to integrate their control into primary health care structures have often not been possible to the desired extent, as these structures have proved to be too feeble. This puts us in the desperate position where such tools as effective vaccines, and important drugs such as Praziquantel and Ivermectine, cannot be delivered to the populations in need. We consider this one of the most urgent problems to be solved. These are instances of the tools being appropriate and highly acceptable, but the resources inadequate.

Similar problems are observed in the control of AIDS, aggravated by the unavailability of treatment. The diagnostic technology alone constitutes a considerable financial and human-resource burden on countries, as the human resources have to be familiarized with advanced immunological techniques. Industries and agriculture have serious effects on health, and occupational health services require technology, first, to diagnose and describe the detrimental effects, and second, to take preventive action. Areas which have attracted little attention in the past are now becoming important, such as waste disposal (including disposable products).

Even the most simple and appropriate technology requires maintenance and repair. Without such services no health service will function. We have therefore begun to train medical technicians in several countries, but also the users of equipment need to be trained. The most difficult task in this context has been to provide spare parts to repair an enormous variety of products donated and bought from all over the world.

Orthopaedic technology is a specialized field that can serve as an example to highlight many of the difficulties involved in determining the appropriate level of technology to be provided for patients. The literature contains examples of the most simple technology, e.g. the use of bamboo to construct primitive appliances. We have chosen to provide essentially the technology used in Europe, however, giving technicians more advanced training so that they can produce most components themselves, even in the poorer countries.

The provision and production of essential drugs is a cornerstone of any health service. The local production of drugs, or at least their formulation, has often been unsuccessful, as production facilities can rarely compete with international suppliers. This prevents the transfer of technologies and raises the question whether the protection of national markets is a worthwhile sacrifice. However, quality control is a must for countries that have to rely on international suppliers. The transfer of technology in this sector may be a prerequisite to ensuring developing countries a fair choice of products, at least.

The provision of modern data-processing equipment was considered until recently a luxury for developing countries. However, as prices have fallen to the level of sophisticated typewriters, even the staunchest critics have become silent. Computers may now be considered an important instance of the significant benefits that a quantum leap in technology may well bestow on even the poorest countries. Obviously they do not have to pass through the same stages of development as the industrialized countries have passed through in the last 50 years.

The laboratory sector technologically is among the most complex sectors. It has therefore also become the most difficult to transfer to developing countries. The preoccupation with the work of village health workers in the last decade has resulted in a certain neglect of laboratories. Probably, too much emphasis was placed on simple clinical diagnosis without the aid of tools, and hence even the microscope was at times forgotten as a powerful diagnostic tool. AIDS has forced upon us the most modern diagnostic technology, and together with similarly powerful methods is again drawing our attention to the medical laboratory.

The technological dilemma in developing countries

Industrialized countries have for long been under the illusion that the best available technology in medical care could be provided to almost the entire population. As costs have skyrocketed and health care consumed a disproportionate share of national income, control measures had to be taken. It has been extremely difficult to find a consensus among professionals on criteria for cutting costs. Some attempts have been made to measure the Quality Adjusted Life Years (QUALY) gained by specific procedures in relation to cost.

Political consensus has been even more difficult to attain, in view of the vested interests of many influential pressure groups, including industry as a key provider of technological tools. The difficulties that industrialized countries meet in balancing the level of desirable technology with affordability, where everybody has access to essential medical care, are almost negligible compared with those of developing countries, where large populations have no access to modern, life-saving medical care.

Technological choices become crucial when expenditure on an X-ray machine has to be weighed against an adequate supply of penicillin to prevent death from pneumonia. If the objective of health services in developing countries is to reduce mortality equitably in as large a population as the financial resources permit, the technological choices would probably need to be reduced to the provision of vaccines, oral rehydration, antibiotics to control death from pneumonia, malaria control, family planning, maternal care and child nutrition, to name the potentially most life-saving technologies. However, it is unrealistic to believe that such a health service would be politically and culturally acceptable.

The reality is that in most developing countries more than 50% of their scarce national resources are spent on national or regional tertiary-care hospitals, which make relatively small contributions to the reduction of those killer diseases. What is normally found is a two-tier system, providing almost industrialized-country standard medical care to a few privileged, mostly urban, populations, while the majority are under-served. Even seriously socialist countries that have attempted to develop more equitable systems have not been able to avoid this dilemma, although the spectrum of equity is broad and some countries have made remarkable progress in the reduction of morbidity and mortality with small national health budgets.

Also, it must be realized that the credibility of the village health worker, who can make a significant contribution to reducing mortality at low cost, is at stake, if he or she cannot refer patients to an appropriate level of referral. National high-income groups, political leaders, foreign residents and tourists also demand sophisticated services, without which neither the nationals nor the foreigners would be likely to stay, but would seek such services in the more advanced countries, with detrimental effects on development.

In their cooperation with developing countries, technical cooperation agencies and donors in general face the same problems and difficult choices, unless they are guided by their national interests alone.

Balancing needs, demand and supply

Some needs can be objectively determined by epidemiological studies. However, felt needs may differ from these very significantly, depending on the social and economic group. It is often these that determine demand, although most countries have opted for a primary health care policy. Demand is frequently also determined by the very serious foreign exchange situation, and requests are submitted for the supply of urgently needed consumable supplies to maintain routine services. Thus precious technical assistance funds are used for the maintenance of services rather than for the transfer of technological expertise.

At the same time, requests are submitted for such advanced technical tools as X-ray machines, computerized tomography (CT) or magnetic resonance images, for which it is difficult to provide technical personnel and operating support. Donors are in a difficult position with regard to making rational decisions. Industry has a strong interest in supplying products and opening up new markets. Representatives of developing countries are often trained in industrialized countries and are very familiar with the technologies available. Politicians are interested in promoting technological advance for their constituencies, and what donor can seriously deny the provision of a technology which is commonplace in his own society without risking the accusation of subscribing to a double ethical standard?

Only a cautious dialogue between representatives from both developing and industrialized countries can bring us closer to solutions that provide for a maximum of equity without excluding the developing countries from technological progress.

Sharing technological progress

As Elliott[1] states, technologies provided must be effective, culturally acceptable, affordable, sustainable locally, not overdependent on external skills, measurable as to their performance and politically responsible. Also, the mere supply of technological tools without the fundamental transfer of technological know-how can only be a second choice and only be justified in the short term. There is the risk of an ever-widening technological gap between the two groups of countries if no serious efforts are made to transfer tools, knowledge and skills in a coordinated and forceful manner. The technology transferred must never be stigma-tized as second-rate. It must be generally accepted that developing countries should have access to the most advanced technologies so long as they meet the above criteria. Modern technologies may at times also be more economical and easier to learn. Critical areas of potential saving in running-costs and foreign exchange should receive special attention.

The transfer of **used equipment** is a common practice but it is usually an ineffective and even expensive strategy. Most well-meaning individuals and institutions are disappointed when their offers are refused. Fortu-nately, donations of drug samples have become rarer, but dental chairs and X-ray equipment are frequently offered. Even if these are repaired and serviced before being transferred, the cost is often higher than that of providing a new apparatus with appropriate technology. The considera-ble costs of transport and reinstallation are usually not considered, quite apart from the fact that any old equipment is more liable to break down. Sometimes equipment is reconditioned in the country of origin, but again the question is whether this is really economical and whether this work should not rather be done in the receiving countries by their own trained technicians. This would mean at least some transfer of skills instead of a marginal employment effect in industrialized countries.

The training of **medical maintenance and repair technicians** is an important first step in transferring technological know-how; it not only prolongs the lifetime of equipment and reduces operating costs but also enables national staff to acquire more advanced technical knowledge and skills. This has to be accompanied by the provision of **spare parts**, which are particularly difficult to obtain because of the diversity of products supplied by donors. Local production of spare parts may be a suitable answer, which at the same time can transform knowledge and skills into sustainable production, and ultimately the development of appropriate technologies. The private sector may play an important role in this context.

A necessary but politically difficult step is the standardization of medical equipment. Donors all too often insist on supplying their own national brands without due consideration of serviceability. At the same time, the markets of developing countries for medical equipment are so small that industry in the other countries probably cannot be persuaded to take account of their special needs. The technology is tailored to profit and to the efficient service networks of industrialized countries. Microscopes could easily be fitted with car bulbs instead of specially fitted products that need to be reordered from the producer. Many firms find it uneconomical to provide service, especially to remote rural areas. On delivery, service manuals are often incomplete or not in the national language, and too few essential spares are provided. There is no point in forcing companies to provide services that do not pay in economic terms, but considerable progress may be made if users are trained to develop suitably standardized specifications and are able to carry out quality control.

A further step towards effective technology transfer may be the development of research and development centres, which could start out by testing the suitability of existing equipment and evaluating user practices and errors, and ultimately prepare their own blueprints. Donors should actively support such developments.

Solar energy converters, both thermal and photovoltaic, are still underused technologies. For new health-service structures solar water-heaters should become standard technology, as equipment can usually be constructed locally and maintenance is minimal. Regrettably, the technology for equipment requiring high temperatures, e.g. sterilizers, is not yet fully developed and is still rather expensive, but for small facilities in remote areas solar technology would be a breakthrough. Photovoltaic technology has the same drawbacks and its application has been limited mostly to lighting and refrigeration. Cost-benefit analysis may have favoured traditional solutions in the past, as the hidden cost of conventional technologies have often not been considered adequately.

Drugs, contraceptive and immunological techniques and genetic engineering may be promising avenues if properly developed. The difficulty is, however, that much of this development is taking place in private industry, with profit as the primary objective. It is therefore important to identify those areas that are not covered by patents and that hold promise of application in the near future.

Potentially cost-saving technologies should be selected, or those that provide better quality at equal cost. Most developments in this area will probably overtax the abilities of individual countries, e.g. in vaccine development or drug production. In addition, the markets may be too small. Only regional efforts are likely to succeed and attract the necessary donor support.

Electronic data-processing equipment is becoming an important asset in health services. It may be used to make more rational management decisions, and can also improve diagnostic and treatment procedures in conjunction with modern communication.

Developing countries urgently need research centres to develop and support the above activities. While there can be no doubt that many such countries already recognize this as a priority, the harsh economic climate is an almost insurmountable hindrance. The salaries offered are totally inadequate to attract young scientists, who often prefer to stay in the industrialized countries where they received their training.

The health sector has suffered more than others from the cuts due to the world economic crisis. Unless health budgets in developing countries are restored to at least pre-crisis level (about 10% of national budgets), the chances of modern technological developments being effectively transferred to developing countries will be minimal, and the gap in the quality of health care between North and South will widen even more.

Reference

[1] Elliott, K. (1984), Appropriate technology (Editorial). *British Medical Journal*, 288: 1251–2.

THE PHARMACEUTICAL INDUSTRY AND HEALTH TECHNOLOGY TRANSFER

R.B. Arnold*

Like so many other terms in common usage, technology transfer has become a jargon catch-phrase. The characteristic of most catch-phrases is that, while they are well known to all individually, it is difficult to attribute to them a precise, universally accepted definition. We all know what we mean by the term but we may not all mean the same thing.

In the context of drugs, I suggest that, when we talk about technology transfer, what we should mean is the transfer of the *benefits* of medicines developed in one country to another country. Although, by definition, the technology will almost certainly be created in an industrialized country, it may be transferred to other industrialized countries as well as developing countries. The range of technology will extend from the drug product itself, which should be regarded as being inseparable from the information on its therapeutic indication(s) and proper use, at one end of the spectrum, to production know-how for the manufacture of intermediates for the drug substance, at the other end. It will include information which has been generated to establish its safety, quality and efficacy, know-how on the manufacture of drug substance, formulation, packaging, plant design and construction, and, most important, test methods and quality-control procedures. At this stage I should point out that my remarks are directed more towards pharmaceuticals than biologicals, although much of what I have to say also applies to the latter.

The process of the clinical evaluation of new drugs should also be viewed as part of the technology-creation process. In the context of developing countries, local clinical trials can produce useful benefits in terms of both the acquired resources, such as hospital equipment, and additional skills and experience of local medical personnel. Perhaps we can regard this as part of the process of information-technology transfer. Of course, clinical trials can range from straightforward user-trials requiring relatively little infrastructure to basic clinical pharmacology, which will need a dedicated hospital unit. And the process can be extrapolated back even further. Just as basic manufacture is the endpoint in production technology transfer, so basic pharmaceutical research can be regarded as the ultimate in information-technology transfer.

If the transfer of technology is to be successful, the receiving environment has to be suitably receptive so that the technology can be fully utilized and products arising from its use are of acceptable and consistent standard and can find a market. I shall expand on some of the economic and practical criteria later on.

---

  * Executive Vice-President, International Federation of Pharmaceutical Manufacturers Associations (IFPMA), Geneva, Switzerland.

Technology transfer will involve one, some, or all of the stages that I have just mentioned but, in my view, has to develop by following a logical sequence (Table 1). Production technology must start with the supply of the finished product together with relevant information on use. Any extension of technology transfer must follow the sequence culminating in basic manufacture. Production technology will require other associated technology for its successful application (Table 2). The evolutionary stages for information technology transfer is shown in Table 3.

Table 1. Stages in technology transfer: Production

- Import of finished product
- Packaging from imported bulk dosage form
- Formulation from imported active ingredient
- Manufacture of drug substance
- Manufacture of intermediates

Table 2. Associated technology required for production technology

- Quality control
  - Pharmaceutical
  - Microbiological/Biological
  - Chemical
- Good manufacturing practice
- Packaging
- Plant design and construction

Table 3. Stages in technology transfer: Information

- Open clinical trials ("User trials")
- Controlled clinical trials
- Clinical pharmacology
- Specific animal studies
- Basic research

What is being discussed today is the transfer of technology from rich to poor countries, not from rich to rich countries. Nevertheless, in the special field of modern medicines no country can hope to be totally self-sufficient. All the industrialized countries, even the industrial giants such as the U.S., Japan and the Federal Republic of Germany, make extensive use of products and technology created in other countries. Apart from the US and Japan, on average, approximately 80% of patent applications in an industrialized country are filed by non-nationals. Any attempt at self-sufficiency in the field of medicines can only be to the detriment of the best interests of the population as a whole, since it will greatly restrict the range, effectiveness and quality of products available to the patient.

For the poorer countries, the acquisition of new technology can occur in three ways:

- by a multinational company setting up or expanding its business in the country;
- by a local entrepreneur acquiring technology by a licensing or purchase arrangement;
- by the intervention of an international agency such as the United Nations Industrial Development Organization (UNIDO) and either government facilities or a local entrepreneur for its application.

Of these three possibilities, the first is believed to offer the best prospect for the acquisition of state-of-the-art technology, for a number of reasons. First, the multinational company will ensure that optimal conditions exist in the receiving country for the use of the technology, which, after all, it has created in the first place. As well as this primary technology, it will include the availability and, if necessary, design and construction of the necessary plant, provision of the associated technology required, including quality control operations, and training of personnel. As a corollary of this there is a greater assurance of the quality of the final product than of that arising through the other channels. International companies operate international quality standards and apply controls to ensure that they are maintained.

Second, the technology available through the other two routes is unlikely to be the most up-to-date. Unless the local licensee has a particularly sophisticated plant and facilities already, he is not going to be able to operate advanced technology to the standards required by a multinational licensor, without very high investment. Technology available from international agencies will, for the most part, have to be acquired from elsewhere by donation or purchase and is likely to relate only to long-established products.

My main thesis today, therefore, is that the most fruitful approach to technology transfer is via the international private-sector pharmaceutical industry and that it is now necessary to look at some of the factors which will encourage this to happen. In passing I would mention that in a few cases international companies have provided viable technology to some international agencies, of which UNIDO is one such, for the manufacture of some long-established products which are nevertheless still extensively used, and which feature in the WHO Model List of Essential Drugs. At that stage, however, the products concerned are unlikely to be of much commercial interest to the originating company because of the large number of competitors.

So what are the factors that will encourage international companies to transfer technology by moving through the sequence of increasing local involvement illustrated in Table 1?

First, if any stage of local manufacture is to be contemplated, the market for the product must be sufficiently large to make it economically viable. This must include possible export as well as domestic sales, but other important criteria must be met if production is envisaged to meet export demands. There is inevitably resistance to imports by one developing country from another, and every country wants to be a net exporter rather than an importer.

Respect for intellectual property is a very important prerequirement for local manufacturing investment by a multinational company, and I would include both patents and trademarks in this term. Not only must enforceable patent protection be available for products as well as processes, but also there should be an adequate period of effective patent life without the threat of compulsory licences. Furthermore, the use of trademarks should be permitted without restriction. It is sometimes suggested that patent protection is a barrier to technology transfer. I would emphatically deny this; indeed the very opposite is the case.

Government pricing policies, where price controls are applied, should be fair and transparent. Risk of sudden arbitrary price cuts, judged from past experience, would be a strongly negative factor.

Government fiscal and import policies must be sympathetic. Import of manufacturing components should not be hampered by exchange control restrictions or excessive duties. The repatriation of reasonable profits should be permitted and taxation should not be at a penal level.

There should be no restrictions on the import of active ingredients, intermediates, and packaging materials or the choice of sources for these components, since such restrictions could be highly prejudicial to the quality of the final product.

The employment of key expatriate staff should be permitted, certainly until suitably qualified local personnel can be found and trained.

Of course, there will be counterbalances to these requirements. The list of reasonable obligations on the part of the company bringing in the technology might be:

- use of local raw materials and packaging, when these are of adequate quality and assured availability;
- maximal employment and training of local staff;
- support for the local health-care infrastructure;
- provision of medicines that are relevant to the health demands and needs of the country.

In my earlier remarks, I rather dismissed the significance of the acquisition of technology in the public sector. Perhaps this is a little unfair, since I recognize that there are, in some countries, public sector production units that are viable and producing products of acceptable quality. However, they are not numerous. A number of countries, however, seem to be attracted by the possibility of their own production resources, in the belief that the drug supply can be improved, and that foreign exchange demands can be diminished and costs reduced. I would offer some words of caution.

In the first place it is necessary to be quite clear as to whether local manufacture is intended to be primarily a health objective or an economic objective. The former implies an attempt to improve the supply to the people of the country of effective medicines of acceptable quality at an affordable price. The second implies concern for foreign exchange flow, employment and the creation of local industry. The two objectives may by no means be compatible. Either way, however, a careful and realistic cost analysis is necessary before a decision is taken.

The acquisition of one or two tabletting machines may be seen as a fairly inexpensive start for a pharmaceutical manufacturing operation. But if generally accepted standards of manufacturing practice and quality are to be met, they may not be used interchangeably for certain types of product such as antibiotics, and must be housed separately. A comprehensive quality-control laboratory will have to be set up, with highly qualified and trained personnel, which will at the same time be heavily under-utilized unless the product range and volume are adequate. Procurement of supplies, allowing for delivery delays and uncertainty, has to be carefully planned and high inventories of some items may have to be accepted to guarantee continuity of production, especially since in many countries most components involved in production will have to be imported. The cost and feasibility of maintenance and repair of equipment must also be considered. The high overheads, if properly costed, can therefore result in a very expensive product, and these factors need to be properly assessed before deciding to embark on public-sector local manufacture.

From the point of view of the local economy, pharmaceutical production involves relatively few people but with a high proportion of qualified staff, whose skills may not be readily available in the country.

I do not want to sound a prophet of doom but, like marriage, pharmaceutical production is not a course of action to be entered into lightly without careful thought of the consequences. Where it can be justified there are significant benefits to be gained from local manufacture, especially when involving a multinational company. These are:

- development of technical and managerial skills by local personnel, which might otherwise be difficult to acquire. This might include support for local academic institutions in providing training in certain disciplines;
- the added value of the goods produced and consequent reduced foreign-exchange requirements;
- possible opportunities for local shareholders. Many international companies have accepted some local investment in their subsidiaries;
- the benefits, perhaps limited, for local peripheral supply industries;
- possible export business.

Before I finish, I should like to revert to the theme of this meeting—whose is the responsibility for the transfer of technology? To a considerable extent I believe that it is not so much a question of responsibility as a natural consequence of a sympathetic and appropriate environment. Imposed obligations against an unsuitable background, with lack of infrastructure and arbitrary government policies, are unlikely to achieve the acquisition which developing countries need. I am reminded of Aesop's fable in which the wind and the sun argued about which could cause a traveller to remove his cloak. The harder the wind blew, the tighter the traveller wrapped his cloak about him. But the sun had only to shine, and off it came straight away. I think there is a lesson to be learned here.

THE RESPONSIBILITY OF THE FIRST-WORLD UNIVERSITY IN HEALTH TECHNOLOGY TRANSFER

P.E.S. Palmer*

I have already prepared two versions of this report: this is the third attempt to answer briefly a very complex set of questions about the responsibility of the university. The first version was written in California, while I was surrounded by every modern technical marvel, both for medical practice and for information retrieval. The second was conceived a few months later in a small country in Africa, where I was surrounded mainly by nature. All I had was a mini-cassette recorder so that my comments could be sent back to be typed in California. I should add that I am equally at home in either situation, for, although I now work at a major Western university, I have spent and still spend a lot of my time in universities and small hospitals in many different parts of the world. I am always intrigued to find how similar are the difficulties and needs, in spite of the wide differences in national preferences and lifestyles.

My first version reflected the surroundings in which it was written and was concerned with the practical aspects of the transfer of technology. In the end the major problem is "money", but there are other considerations worth exploring. Amongst these is the basic choice that must be made: "Where should the transfer, the teaching and learning take place?". This is not too difficult to answer. In most cases it will be easier and more productive for the transfer of high technology to begin where there is every facility, background information and a support group of graduate and undergraduate students. The students will provide stimulation, and there will be other, interrelated departments to provide more information. Of course, there will later have to be proper follow-up in the new surroundings of the recipient country.

For complex technology, it is clear that the transfer is a multi-layered task. It should start in the provider university, with the education of colleagues or graduate students from the recipient country, who even at this stage should give their own views as to what part of the technology may later need modification. Changes are better made before transfer, not in the less-equipped surroundings of the new country.

This is particularly true of medical techniques and technology: the pattern of disease, the social awareness of patients, the other equipment available and the outlook of the local medical community will influence the way in which patients are treated and thus the way in which new technology is used. Teacher and student will have to work together, learning from each other until together they have produced the correct solution for that country or, in some instances, for that part of the country. In my experience the commonest error is for both sides to

---

* Professor, Department of Radiology, University of California, Davis, California, USA.

underestimate the difficulties of the transfer and overestimate its impact. Seldom will they correctly guess how long it will take.

If visitors are to be brought from one country to another, the practical side cannot be forgotten. Failure to get the "paperwork" organized in advance can waste valuable time, energy and money. The university must provide administrative support services, with knowledge of local requirements for visas, work permits, housing and any liability for taxation. Included where appropriate should be health insurance and simple practical information such as maps of the town and of bus and other transport routes, campus and library rules, how to make copies, where to eat, and where to get advice on anything. A large university can be a bewildering place, and support should include more than money. This is also true for the teacher going to the recipient country, who will often need not only the above information but also warnings, in some countries, about dress codes and local customs. A social gaffe may not only hinder the technological transfer but also have dire personal consequences. An alcoholic drink, a polite smile at someone's wife, failure to bring a gift or giving a gift with the wrong hand may, at the very least, lower the credibility of the visiting expert.

Other speakers will discuss that word which is missing from the lexicon of so many developing countries, "maintenance". While this is not a prime university responsibility, it is irresponsible of any university to recommend or facilitate the transfer of any technology—or technique—that cannot be sustained. It cannot be shrugged off as being outside the university's terms of reference.

With regard to less complex technology, or to techniques, then I am from my own experience biased against bringing individuals to learn, in the hope that they will return to spead the knowledge. On the practical side there is usually a significant time needed to adjust to living in a different context, and such time is unproductive. There are also likely to be so many other things of interest, not all academic or technical, that the visitor is distracted from the main purpose. I do not deny the enormous benefits of wider education and general knowledge, but we are discussing the transfer of technology, not broadening someone's background, which usually takes much longer. When research is involved there must be case-by-case, practical judgment. It may be better started at the provider university, but my own bias favours carrying out research wherever the outcome will be used.

When considering an invitation to a colleague to come and learn at an established centre, we cannot overlook the fact that, on return, there will be undeniable limitations on any prophet in his or her own country. However reliable the prophecies, they will seldom be heeded as well as those that come with the aura of elsewhere. The expert and strange teacher can be a magnet to attract many unbelievers.

Many universities maintain "outreach" offices. For example, the University of California has offices in Nairobi, Cairo, Paris, Lyons and elsewhere. These were started to help students on elective courses, both those coming to the different country and those who wish to study in California. Much more use should be made of these widely established centres, even to the extent, if necessary, of asking for help from another university when technology transfers are contemplated or take place. A clearing-house should be established, either at such centres or in the recipient university (or perhaps at the WHO country office) where at least basic information on all current collaborative research projects and technical transfers should be available. Much overlap could be prevented: the unexpected need for additional expertise with one project might be met by another expert carrying out some other transfer. While visiting one country for WHO recently I was able to help and became involved in another WHO project just when expert advice was needed and was not locally available. This was by chance: it would be very useful if there were a continually updated list of what expertise was locally available, kept locally by WHO or in a university office? At such offices it should also be possible to obtain immediate help when any local tradition or deeply ingrained custom may be at cross-purposes with the new technology. Tradition cannot be ignored; it may arise from very valid local reasons. The university is the proper source of guidance, and everyone should know where to find help.

If visiting teachers are sent to other universities to establish new ideas and new techniques as well as new technologies, time should be available so that they are not overwhelmed by their direct teaching responsibilities. They must be able to adapt to the way their students think, to local values, ideas and concerns. Only in this way can technology not only be transferred but also be accepted.

Having dealt with the question " where should transfer take place? " I went on to the next: who leads the process of transfer? This cannot be delegated to the least experienced on the grounds that the project is straightforward and all problems have been anticipated so that anyone can carry on. This is never true. There will always be unexpected hitches, some difference needed in technique or approach, some outcome to be analysed and put into the local context. For these reasons the teacher must be the most experienced available, which usually means someone senior (but not always!). When they have to go abroad, it has been argued, they will be missed at home. However, often there is a team at the provider-university that can do the job perfectly well, whereas more than technical knowledge is needed when ideas and technology are to be transferred elsewhere. The choice of who is to go must be made very carefully: the assignment seldom turns out to be a relaxing few weeks in exotic surroundings. Enormous tact is almost always essential: dogma and superiority will be resented. Technology must be physically and philosophically fitted into its new surroundings, neither dumped nor forcibly stuffed into place. The teacher—a composite term for all the responsibilities inherent in transferring technology—should be confident and relaxed, know the job, be able to communicate and contribute at any level, and be willing to change the approach as the situation demands. Merely knowing how to screw the parts together and press the required buttons is but a very small part of technology transfer. Of course, I have ignored the basic question as to whether the technology should be there at all: by now it is too late and for better or worse that decision has been made!

It was at this stage here that the second version of my paper was born. After visiting again three countries in Africa I came up against some broad ethical questions, which in California had appeared simple to answer, or overlook. I almost completely re-wrote my contribution.

It would seem that everyone would agree that any technology to be transferred should:

- be of practical use to the country concerned;
- be capable of reliable and cost-efficient functioning;
- serve the majority of the people, at reasonable cost.

What happens in practice is not so straightforward.

I had been asked to advise on the development of imaging services at all levels throughout the country. The solutions were really very straightforward and, to me, as obvious as the needs: not the blanket importation of all I had left in California, but a selection of equipment and training programmes which, while technically advanced, would provide what was needed locally for their health services. Of course, the main barrier was "money", this time complicated by politics. Both were present but, for me, in the wrong proportions. Because of what I have termed "politics" in a very broad sense, money was short.

To make matters worse, commerce had already "transferred" technology (at a price) and taken unfair advantage of the complete absence of expert knowledge locally. Technically outdated and unsuited items had been sold, presumably because there were few other places which would accept them. Some had even been mislabelled as being the WHO-specified Basic Radiological System, and had been accepted in good faith by the authorities because of that assurance. This tactic is not new in history. Many a gullible owner has been sold a phoney racehorse. Imaging equipment is expensive and, like any racehorse, costly to maintain, and can easily run away with the budget.

How was I to deal ethically with this situation? In the end I fell back on the general principle that a university professor has no right to suppress knowledge, and I shall come back to that later. In Africa my frustration was increased by the fact that the country had been offered a gift of a computerized tomography (CT) scanner. One may compare this with Eve and her apple: in neither case were the ensuing costs and complications properly explained to the recipient. Nor had it been mentioned that at present most of the people in that country could not have a chest X-ray when they needed one.

During this CIOMS meeting I have been interested to see that the advanced technology for imaging disease has caught the imagination and is being referred to by others as an example of desirable technology. The glamour of magnetic resonance imaging, computerised tomography and lithotripsy is easily understood. Glamour often disguises the truth. My department in California is well supplied with CT scanners, MRI, Colour Doppler ultrasound, digitalised this and microchipped that. Our annual departmental budget probably exceeds that for health care in many small countries. This does not mean that our imaging facilities are necessarily used wisely. Glamour can hypnotise any physician, and a

$ 1000 examination may be used to learn what could just as easily have been found out by using eyes and hands. Universities are not meeting their responsibilities there either!

What must not be overlooked is how few patients benefit from this superb technology. There are not many common diseases that can only be diagnosed by MRI, and, of those that can be, many turn out to be incurable even when every specialist skill is also available. CT scanners have much wider use, but need to be put in perspective. My department in California imaged over 140,000 patients last year. Less than 5% had MR or CT, and none was refused because of inability to pay. Research in USA has shown that only about 20% of all patients who undergo CT scanning receive any benefit, judged by a change, or a decision to make no change, in their treatment. Thus, at a generous estimate, less than 2% of patients at a university medical centre benefitted from a capital expenditure of over 5 million US dollars. (Even if the figures are overly conservative, the message is unchanged.) This cost does not include the salaries of technical and specialist staff, running costs and the maintenance of the high technology. In the African country concerned there are no specialists, such as neurosurgeons, on whom the successful treatment of the CT-diagnosed diseases largely depends. The yield from the free CT scanner, if it could be staffed and maintained in operation, would be even lower. No wonder I was frustrated!

Others have referred to lithotripsy. It, too, is a good example of how universities often fail to match and equitably balance the outpourings of the media and of commerce. Make no mistake, ministries of health usually learn of new technology from salesmen or, perhaps even more dificult to evaluate, from specialists who have seen new technology in some other country and return demanding the same facilities for their patients. Neither the salesmen nor the specialists are likely to enthusiastically list the disadvantages, costs and other negative attributes of the equipment they want to sell. This is true of lithotrypsy.

Renal lithotripsy has been successfully used on a small proportion of urinary calculi for some years. A recent symposium at the National Institute of Health showed that it is not free of harmful after-effects in some patients. Similar technology is now available for gallstones, but, unfortunately, at present is suitable for only about 20% of patients with cholelithiasis. One treatment may not suffice: some patients need several sessions. Some patients have complications needing immediate surgery. We do not yet know whether there are any long-term effects, but given the nature of the disease some patients are likely to have recurrent stones. Many patients, even when successfully treated, need drug therapy for some months afterwards. If only 20% of patients are suitable, it means that to treat two patients a day (which is not cost-efficient) the hospital or clinic will have to see 10 new patients with gallstones every day. If there are so many patients there is need for an epidemiological survey and public-health measures aimed at prevention! And gallstone lithotripsy must be evaluated in comparison with well-established surgery, which has a low complication rate, can remove all the stones at once and ensures that there is no underlying tumour. Even if low-cost lithotripsy becomes available, it will need much more experience before it becomes a practical replacement for surgeons in remote places, or even in major centres.

I have discussed these very expensive and complex technologies because other speakers at this round-table conference have referred to them. Well, they do demonstrate some of the difficulties! They are, in many ways, miraculous and there is an overwhelming desire for miracles in health care, but they show clearly the need for caution and very careful investigation before accepting miracles into everyday use. Far too many technologies are introduced into our industrialized medical world without proper evaluation. They may indeed perform well and do all that is claimed, but is the benefit real, are they really needed, are they cost-efficient? Are they applicable and affordable in every community? Who will work them? Above all, will they help many people without adversely affecting other important programmes?

Clearly the universities, together with WHO, must accept the responsibility for dispassionate assessment. Perhaps even more important, it is the responsibility of the universities to teach attitudes. Very few medical schools train students to recognize or judge when technology is appropriate or when its use is not necessary. The constant demand is for more and more, without proper regard to benefit and with even less regard to cost. Our colleagues, the physicians and health officials of non-industrialized countries, pay us visits, read medical journals and believe that this is the way that medicine *must* be practised, that no other way is acceptable. Universities have the responsibility to teach values, in medicine as in everything else, *not* only "how to" do something but also to discuss benefits and disadvantages.

Unfortunately it is often technology and commerce, *not* the university, that tell us what is now needed or what we should think is needed. Universities must open minds, not only books, so that decisions can be made independently of whether the technology is there or not. Not everything that comes from a computer is true. We apply that principle when we look at our bank accounts or credit-card records, but too frequently fail to apply it to medicine. We need to ask questions, cynically and with enquiring, doubting, minds until we are convinced by the answers. Do we need it, will our patients benefit, can they afford it, can they do without it, and, perhaps most important, will they really suffer if that technology is not there? Every medical journal and professional or technical publication should include a complete list of complications, costs, disadvantages and hangovers.

High technology needs more than specifications. Like surgery, there should be informed consent from the recipient before it is transferred.

So much for the first two versions of this report: was there any overlap? Yes, on the question of ethics, because ultimately technology transfer is a practical problem that can be solved in many ways and, given good will on both sides, with satisfactory results. It is in the ethics of transfer that there are difficulties.

Neither in California nor in Africa did I have any real doubt that knowledge must be transferred freely and openly. It can only be equally shared. I do not believe that anyone will seriously disagree with that, or with the premise that all knowledge on any subject must be given, nothing hidden or suppressed, whether we personally believe it is good or bad. We cannot set ourselves up as both teachers and judges. We may, and should, express doubts, enthusiasm and opinions, and stimulate debate formed on information, but we cannot take decisions on behalf of anyone else. We are not superior, but simply at times more fortunate.

Nor can a university be over-concerned with commerce, although business interests will affect much that may or may not happen. If a drug, technique or equipment is to be used on man by man, then every aspect of its effect and constituents must be made known to those who want to use it, without regard to commercial interests or patents. Perhaps we should include here the university's attitude to the threat of legal action (malpractice) if all does not go according to plan. This is covered by the concept that the university has the responsibility to make all information known openly to everyone concerned. Clearly the threat of lawsuits will affect governmental regulations in many countries. It is not satisfactory to apply blindly the rules of one country to another: local conditions must be taken into consideration, and the university may be the proper place for reassessment of imported or exported regulations for technology.

There is another major question of principle that must be considered: does a university have to wait to be asked or should it take active steps when there is a new technology that will be of use to another country? My personal view is that it is very much the responsibility of a university to pass on information not only in the usual way, by journal publications and professional congresses, but also with the help of organizations such as WHO. One of the major difficulties in the developing world is to know what information is already available, what technology has been developed or where to get it. The African country offered a CT scanner did not know that there is a WHO scientific report providing not only specifications but also a clear opinion on what else is needed before a CT scanner can be justified, what costs would be involved in installation and maintenance and who would benefit[1]. From this report a decision could have been made on the basis of knowledge. There is so far a failure to transmit information as well as technology, and this is a very urgent problem, which needs to be addressed.

If all the already available technology for health care were put into use, health services would be very different. However, they would not necessarily be better in every way, for there is that difficult-to-define but universally recognized aspect of knowledge and informed choice, which is essential if the technology is to play its part properly and not merely be an exciting, novel and fashionable gadget. Universities have a major role to play in guiding these choices, because the knowledge they provide should, above all, be impartial and without vested interest.

How, in practice, can universities and WHO provide more guidance? There are an increasing number of organizations providing scientific or technical assessment reports; there is even an association of such organizations. Too often, however, they do not provide an opinion. They say whether the machine works but not whether it is ideal for a specific situation. To take a simple example: X-ray equipment should be chosen after considering not only what needs to be X-rayed, but also who is going to use it: a trained radiographer or an inexperienced operator? Of course, this is but one factor affecting the decision, but it is a vital consideration. Universities should be prepared to advise, which in most cases means that somebody has to go to the recipient country, visit the hospitals, talk to local doctors and, I fear, local politicians as well as health administrators, and try to assess the impact of the technology as well as the more simple question of whether it will work. Nowhere is there enough money to provide health care on the basis of what is new and fashionable, a message which must be continuously broadcast.

Finally, the most vexed ethical question of all: How do universities, or in practice their representatives in the field, react when some decision is, by all normal standards (not just their own), not in the best interests of the whole community? By using the local media? This is, perhaps, unethical, and if the local press is government-controlled it may backfire. Telling the ministry concerned may not work if it is the pet project of a major politician. Attacking the donor country often fails, as the choice is so often blamed on the recipient country, while the provider claims that "interference in the affairs of another country is not possible" (A strange viewpoint if your gift is about to disrupt the economy). Into many such situations come the complicating factors of ego, pride, prestige and keeping up with the neighbours.

Sometimes the problem has arisen simply from lack of information. Information is easily supplied and, once this has been done, anything else may be interpreted as interference, causing resentment and lack of credibility. When this happens the argument is already lost.

Here none of my three versions comes up with a satisfactory answer, and I cannot separate my instincts from my opinions. This is where CIOMS needs to provide guidance to universities and similar advisory bodies. All other responsibilities dissolve into practical ways and means, subject to argument as to which is best, but usually working anyway despite the many differing approaches. While delving into the ethics and upheavals of exotic technology we cannot forget that, in over half the world, when one's leg is broken it cannot be X-rayed. No CT scanner, MRI, PET scanner, or ultrasound will help, even if there happens to be one around the corner. Most of us break legs or suffer from straightforward curable diseases rather than obscure tumours. Moreover, we face most of the manageable illnesses when we are young and vital members of the community, when failure to heal or recover affects many others as well as the individual patient.

The Chairman has asked us to mention some successful technology. Continuing in the same theme of broken legs and needed chest X-rays, there is the WHO Basic Radiological System (BRS). This is a highly sophisticated yet very simple to operate X-ray unit, which can be installed and will work almost anywhere. It will examine 95% of all the imaging needs of small hospitals and clinics in rural or suburban settings. It is well-tested in the field and there are over 750 working world-wide. Indeed it could carry out 80 % of the examinations done at a university hosptial without loss of quality. Everywhere it goes it is successful: why has it not gone everywhere? Because the price is kept artificially high by the manufacturers, who require four or three times its real cost, even allowing for a reasonable profit margin. The same design is supplied in large numbers to armed services, but cannot be afforded to meet the needs of the common man. This is another question, both practical and ethical, that needs to be addressed.

Given money, many health-care problems can be solved, but, given money, how can we be sure it is wisely used? Not even the resources of the University of California or the needs of that African country have enabled me to answer that question.

I sincerely hope that I will find the answer here, at CIOMS and WHO, Geneva.

Reference

1 WHO Technical Report Series, NO. 723, 1985 (*Future use of new imaging technologies in developing countries*: report of a WHO Scientific Group).

THE ROLE OF RESEARCH AND SERVICE INSTITUTIONS IN HEALTH TECHNOLOGY TRANSFER

Shigekoto Kaihara*

1. Introduction

I do not know whether there is any accepted definition of *Research and Service Institution*. I have assumed that this is an institution whose main objectives are to conduct health-related research and to provide some kind of health-related scientific service to its country or region.

I come from a university, but I am in charge of a hospital computer centre of the university. Although it is part of a university, its main role is to provide information-processing facilities and services to our university personnel as well as to the national universities all over the country. Therefore, I think it may be included in the category of research and service institutions. First, I shall discuss our experiences in relation to technology transfer, and later I shall try to generalize from the lessons we have learned.

2. Experiences at Hospital Computer Centre, University of Tokyo

Although the main activities of the Hospital Computer Centre are to provide services to hospitals and to teach medical students, it has been active in technology transfer as a WHO collaborating centre. For instance, it has accepted fellows from developing countries and sometimes participated in a project in a developing country.

From these experiences, my present feeling is that technology transfer is a very complicated process, about which it is difficult to generalize. Let me give you some examples. A government employee in a developing country stayed with us for six months. She had been awarded a fellowship and she wanted to learn information-processing in health. At that time, in her country, there was a plan to use computer technology in the statistical processing of health data, and this was one of the reasons she was sent to our centre. She was a very intelligent girl and tried very hard to learn. But the problem was that she did not know what kind of technology she had to learn and what kind of role she was expected to play on return to her country. Information processing in health uses many different levels of technology, and no one person can learn all of them. For instance, anyone who must buy equipment must know the characteristics of various types of computer, and anyone who operates equipment must learn how to operate a specific model of computer.

---

* Professor, Hospital Computer Centre, University of Tokyo, Tokyo, Japan.

These two functions are totally different and usually performed by different sections of an organization. In this case, the government official who sent this young woman to our centre was to blame. He knew that he had to computerize the activities of his section, but he himself did not understand the field and he instructed her only to go to Japan and to learn about computers. She, on her own decision, learned more detailed techniques in Japan, namely computer programming, and returned to her country with excellent skills in computer programming. Some time later, I heard that she was dissatisfied because she could not use what she had learned, and later again, that she had left government service to be employed by a private company at a far higher salary.

In another case, we received two fellows from a hospital in a developing country, which was to instal a computer, and one fellow was supposed to become a systems engineer, and the other a programmer. The computer had not been installed when they left for Japan, so they did not know what size of computer they had to use in the future, and what kinds of applications were to be installed. The planning of a computer system depends very closely on the size and type of computer. The programming language or data-base system are also dependent on a machine. Our fellows did not have this information, so they were given more general training, using the machine available in Japan. The training itself was very successful, but two years after they returned home their hospital installed a computer system totally different from the machine on which they had learned. They had to be trained again. In this case, since I was a member of the Japanese coordinating committee to the hospital, I tried to persuade the funding agency to instal a more common computer, but the decision was made by a different section, independently.

There are some successful cases. Our university department of bio-chemistry received a lady biochemist from a developing country, whose objective was to be trained in a diagnostic molecular-biology method of typing typhoid bacilli. She had been well trained in her discipline and she had planned what she was to do in Japan before she came. Although she stayed only three months, she almost completed what she had set out to do and after her return she set up the new technologies in her laboratory to continue her work.

3. Series of activities for successful transfer of technology

From these experiences, it may be concluded that for the successful transfer of technology the following series of activities must be well coordinated. Ideally the research institutions conduct all these steps, but in reality it is usually not possible.

(a) To make a survey of the health problems as well as the social and economic problems of the developing country and make a strategic plan for solving them.
(b) To determine what technologies are needed to solve the problems.
(c) To help the counterpart to find funds to transfer the technologies.

(d) To train the staff of the counterpart institute in the use of the technologies to be transferred.

(e) To send long-term and short-term consultants to the counterpart institute for follow-up.

(f) To make an assessment of the transferred technologies after the transfer has been completed.

In the first case described above, the technologies needed to solve the problems had not been clearly enough determined, because the survey of the environment had not been made before the fellow came for training. In the second case, coordination with the funding organization was lacking: it made its decision independently of the people on site. In the third case, the people in the counterpart country had completed all the necessary preliminary stages for technology transfer, and only the last step was necessary for its success.

4. The limitations of present research and service institutions

Although ideally the institutions conduct all the steps described above according to need, only few institutions can play such roles. The reality may be as follows:

(a) Ordinary institutions have no personnel to share with developing countries. Their personnel are busy with their daily institutional functions.

(b) Even when the required technologies are identified, the institutions do not have them. The technologies of developing countries are different from these of industrialized countries.

(c) Since the funding organizations and research institutions are not well coordinated, it is difficult to help the counterpart institution find funds.

(d) The institutes have no suitable training courses in the technologies of developing countries.

(e) Consultants to be sent from the institutes may not be familiar with the conditions of the developing countries.

(f) For assessment, there is no standard generally accepted method of technology transfer.

5. What can the institution do?

In spite of the limitations described above, national research and service institutions can contribute to technology transfer if they make some efforts. Their roles would be: 1) to pool various technologies to be transferred; 2) to pool consultants; 3) to conduct training; 4) and to conduct research into the technologies for developing countries. Some factors are especially important if an institution is to be successful and a key place in technology transfer.

5.1. Two types of technology

There are two types of health technology: that designed to identify and prioritize health problems, and that which can be applied in the solution of various health problems. An example of the first type is the technology for making a survey of health problems in a region, and an example of the second is the technology for the immunization of children. When we talk of technology transfer we tend to talk of the second type, but without the first type technology transfer can not be successful. However, the first type must be developed in the receiving country itself: it is extremely difficult if not impossible to transfer it from an industrialized country.

5.2. National Essential Technologies

Although developed countries have so many sophisticated technologies, most are not only unnecessary but also sometimes harmful to developing countries. If each country were to designate the technologies that it finds essential, in the same way as countries have designated essential drugs, the transfer of technology would become less complicated and much easier. I would propose that each developing country designate its *national essential technologies*.

5.3. Complex of sub-technologies

Very often technologies are a set of sub-technologies, and different organizations possess the different sub-technologies. Some may be the property of industries. I recall the story of a man who lived in the desert, totally separate from the civilized world. He was once invited to a city in civilized country. He was impressed especially by the abundance of water, but in general did not like the city life and decided to go back to the desert. His host offered as a gift whatever he wanted. After some thought he said he would like to take back a water faucet, "because I can get water just by twisting it".

This may seem a funny story, but there are many such cases in technology transfer. If only part of the system is transferred, it does not work. In the transfer of such technologies, the availability of all the sub-technology units must be secured by coordinating the contributions of different sectors.

5.4. Technologies for developing countries

From another point of view, technologies may be classified into three types: those that can be applied in developing countries without any modification; those that can be developed by customizing existing technologies to the needs and conditions of developing countries; and those that are applicable only in developing countries.

Usually, research and service institutions in developed countries have only the first type, but developing countries often need the second and third types. This gap must be filled; some effort must be made to develop the second and third type in research and service institutions.

5.5. Specialists in development
Technology transfer cannot be handled together with the daily activities of research institutions of industrialized countries. These institutions must have a small number of specialists in the *management of development* to ensure the success of technology transfer.

5.6. Increase in the institutional capacity of the developing country
The institutional capacity of the counterpart to accept the technologies is the key factor in the successful transfer of technology. Even when all the above factors are provided, if the counterpart in the developing country is unable to analyse the problem and to apply the transferred technologies, the transfer will be sure to fail.

6. Conclusion

In conclusion, the research and service institutions of industrialized countries can become centres for technology transfer, but to do so their present problems and limitations must be realized and some efforts made to lead them in such a direction. For this I recommend that:

(1) research and service institutions acquire the means and skills for coordinating the various sectors of technology transfer, including funding organizations;
(2) research and service institutions set up small units consisting of specialists in the management of development; and
(3) developing countries set up counterpart groups that can analyse problems and manage the process of applying new technologies to their solution.

DEVELOPING-COUNTRY ECONOMISTS AND HEALTH TECHNOLOGY TRANSFER

Kong-Kyun Ro*

1. Introduction: Transfer of Health Technology and General Technology and its Contribution to National Development

There is quantitative and qualitative growth in a nation's economy. The absolute size of a nation's gross national product (GNP) reflects both quantitative and qualitative growth. More people, more physical capital and the resulting increased output represent quantitative growth. Qualitative growth represents increase in productivity, namely more output per worker and per item of equipment.

Technological progress has been the prime source of qualitative growth and the basis of industrial revolution. Innovations during the past two decades have dramatically increased the quantity and quality of output per worker and item of equipment. We have witnessed a vast improvement in the living standards of the developed and newly industrializing countries.

For developing countries, technological transfer has played a greater role than innovations in increasing productivity. Therefore, it is essential for the economic development of developing countries that they receive appropriate technological transfer.

There are three main categories of general technological progress: labour-saving (capital-using), capital-saving (labour-using) and neutral technological advances. Labour-saving technological progress improves labour productivity and tends to use capital-intensive production processes. Capital-saving progress does the opposite. Neutral advances usually improve both labour and capital productivity without changing the labour-capital mix of the production process (Figure 1).

Therefore, labour-saving technological advances benefit mainly labour-scarce economies, and capital-saving advances benefit labour-surplus economies. This leads to mainly capital-saving technology transfer to developing countries with surplus labour and underemployment problems. Labour-saving technology transfer is mainly for relatively more developed countries with labour shortage.

Regardless of the type of technological transfer, the objective is to utilize relatively more abundant resources to improve labour and/or capital productivity for economic growth. Such technological transfer would enable the technology importer to compete better in international trade by strengthening each importing country's comparative advantage.

* Professor, Korea Advanced Institute of Science and Technology, Seoul, Korea.

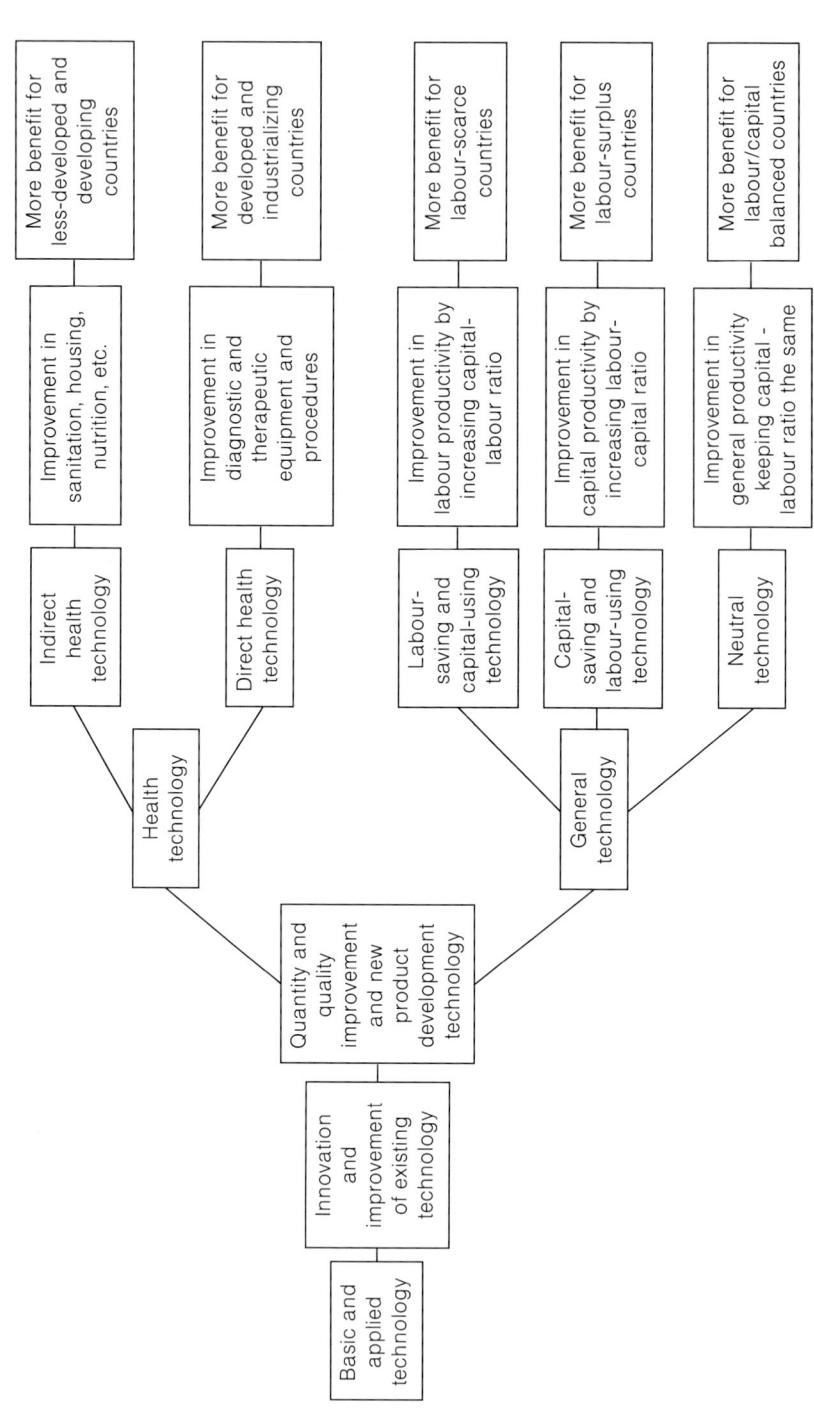

Figure 1. *Health-technology and general-technology transfer compared*

92

Health technology may be broadly divided into two categories: indirect and direct. Indirect health technology is mainly for improving sanitation, housing and nutrition. Import of such technology is given more priority by less developed countries with a weak socioeconomic infrastructure.

Direct health technology is mainly for improving diagnostic and therapeutic procedures and equipment. Recently there has been an impressive advance in direct health technology in the developed countries and in some newly industrializing countries. It has contributed greatly to improving health and human capital and to accelerating national development.

Some, perhaps most, advanced direct health technology is expensive to acquire and to use appropriately. Therefore, extreme caution has to be exercised in the transfer of highly sophisticated health technology. Certain conditions must be met prior to the transfer of advanced technology from developed to less-developed countries.

These are that the receiving country must: 1) be able to absorb the technology; 2) have the technological capability to develop its own technology on the basis of the imported technology; and 3) have a socio-economic infrastructure that can continue to absorb the imported technology and to develop its own technological basis. For transfer of health technology the receiving country must first ensure as a policy priority that it does not import highly sophisticated equipment for only a few privileged people while the rest of the population does not have access to primary health care, and the exporting country must take into consideration this question of equity.

Countries that export and import health technology should assume a greater degree of responsibility than that involved in the transfer of general technology. A strong partnership based on mutual enlightened self-interest has to be established for health-technology transfer to contribute to improving a nation's health, human capital and development.

2. Transfer of General and Health Technology: Similarities and Differences

The basic difference between general and health technology transfer is that the purpose of the former is to increase productivity (output per worker), whereas that of the latter is to improve the quality of output. For both diagnostic and therapeutic health services, the impact of technology has been mainly to improve the quality of care, not to increase the number of cases treated per man-hour. Another difference is that, whereas the purpose of both is to improve quality of life of the recipient countries, the former is designed to do so by increasing material wealth, and the latter by improving health, a prerequisite to the enjoyment of material wealth.

The most important difference is that health technology transfer enables a nation to improve its human capital qualitatively and quantitatively. The improvement in human capital has secondary and tertiary effects: it improves the quality of labour, thereby increasing the worker's production efficiency; and it improves consumption efficiency, thereby enabling the consumer to get more (utility) out of a given consumption (activities).

A similarity of general and health technology transfer is that each improves the receiving country's labour productivity and, in most cases, its technological capability to develop further its own technology (Figure 2).

3. Health and Human Capital

The quality of human capital is now widely recognized as the major factor contributing to national development. Development strategists have shifted their emphasis in investment from physical capital to human capital for achieving sustained economic growth. The late Nobel Laureate, Simon Kuznets, estimated that from 40 to 60% of economic growth in the developed and newly industrializing economies is attributable to investment in human capital. Regrettably, discussion about investment in human capital has been confined mostly to educational capital and knowledge embodied in population. Theodore W. Schultz, another Nobel Laureate and founder of the concept of human capital, stated that "by concentrating on education, we are in danger of losing sight of other sources of human capital". The other or twin source of human capital is health.

Economists tend to consider human capital as the product of joint inputs, namely health and education. Health improves human capital directly by improving the quality of labour, and indirectly by enabling it to achieve a higher level of education. A healthy child is more likely to do school-work better than an ailing child. Just as a nation with a pool of high-quality human capital is better able to absorb technology transfer, a healthy person is better able to absorb knowledge at school and elsewhere.

From this perspective, the success of transfer of appropriate health technology not only contributes to the improvement of human welfare more directly than does transfer of general technology, but also lays a foundation for increasing labour productivity on a more sustained basis.

Going one step further, advances in health technology not only lay a more solid and sustainable foundation for economic growth than does general technological progress, but also set in motion a positive circle of cumulative effects. The contribution of successful transfer of health technology, both directly and indirectly, is that national development takes on a life of its own. As the investment in human capital increases economic growth, more resources become available and are invested further in human as well as physical capital. This, in turn, further accelerates economic growth. This sets in motion a positive circle, thus

94

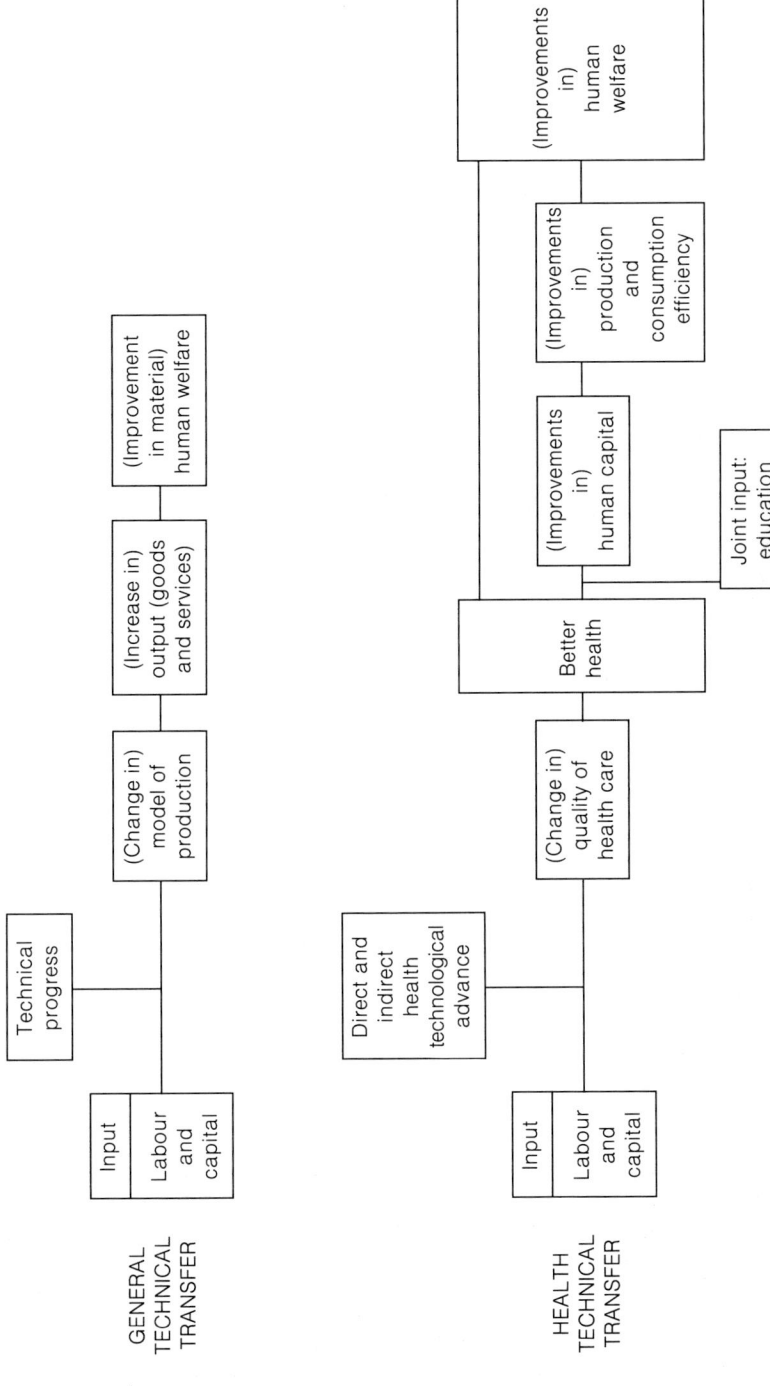

Figure 2. *General-technology and health-technology transfer and their economic impact*

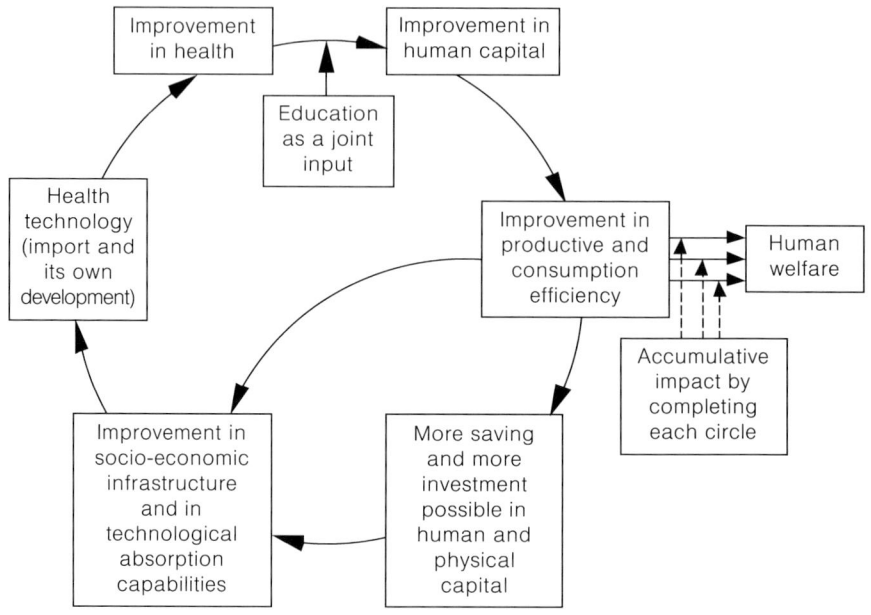

Figure 3. *Advances in health technology and their cumulative effects*

enabling a nation to reach the so-called take-off point in economic growth (Figure 3).

Once this is recognized, the issue is, not whether transfer of health technology is important for national development, but, rather, what factors determine the extent of success of health technology transfer in improving a nation's health and thereby its human capital. For economists the issue is, then, a matter of prioritizing investment options among various kinds of health-technology transfer according to the conditions and circumstances of recipient countries.

4. Selectivity in Health Technology Transfer and Investment Theory

According to investment theory, decisions on kinds of physical capital and amount of investment should be made on the basis of estimated return, cost and the time it will take for the expected yield to materialize. Priority is to be given to the kind of physical capital which is estimated to yield the maximum rate of return among all available investment opportunities.

The kind of health technology to be imported should be decided according to the same criterion. For given infrastructure and technological absorption capabilities, each recipient country should import health technology which is estimated to have the maximum sustained beneficial impact on the nation's health with given expenditure of resources.

Another important factor in selecting health technology to be imported is the estimated period during which the imported technology is to contribute to the nation's health and technological capability, directly and indirectly. For example, in the short run, investment in the transfer of indirect health technology may yield a higher dividend for the less developed countries. Investment in sanitation, housing and nutrition, for example, would improve the nation's health more than investment in state-of-the-art health technology. The resulting improvement in human capital would contribute directly to national development by increasing labour productivity.

In the long run, however, investment in the import of direct appropriate health technology may yield a higher dividend, as import of successful direct health technology would improve the nation's technological capability. This would enable the recipient nation to develop its own general as well as health technology. The development of general technological capability would contribute to national development directly and, by enabling the nation to absorb further general and health technology transfer, indirectly.

Without regard to short- or long-run impact, some less developed countries may find it necessary to import indirect health technologies immediately, because otherwise the nation may not come to possess human resources capable of later absorbing direct health technology.

Beyond the broad question of choosing between indirect and direct health technology, all investments in technology expected to improve any available input for promoting health should be decided according to the investment criterion discussed above. This requires that all inputs that promote health should be examined as to the amount of the marginal contribution they make to health and to their cost.

This, in turn, requires a vast amount of information. As in selecting the optimum portfolio of investments for national development, each developing country's infrastructure, human resources and associated factors would determine the optimum mix of direct and indirect health technology to be imported, and of different kinds and levels of technology to be included in the direct or indirect technology to be imported.

5. Health Technology Import and Optimum Resource Allocation

The ultimate objective of importing either health or general technology is to improve human welfare as much as the given expenditure of resources permits. From the economist's perspective, this objective can be achieved effectively when the import of health technology contributes to the optimum allocation of the nation's limited resources. This indicates that decisions about the kinds of health technology to import are connected with decisions about the amount of money to be spent for ends other than health.

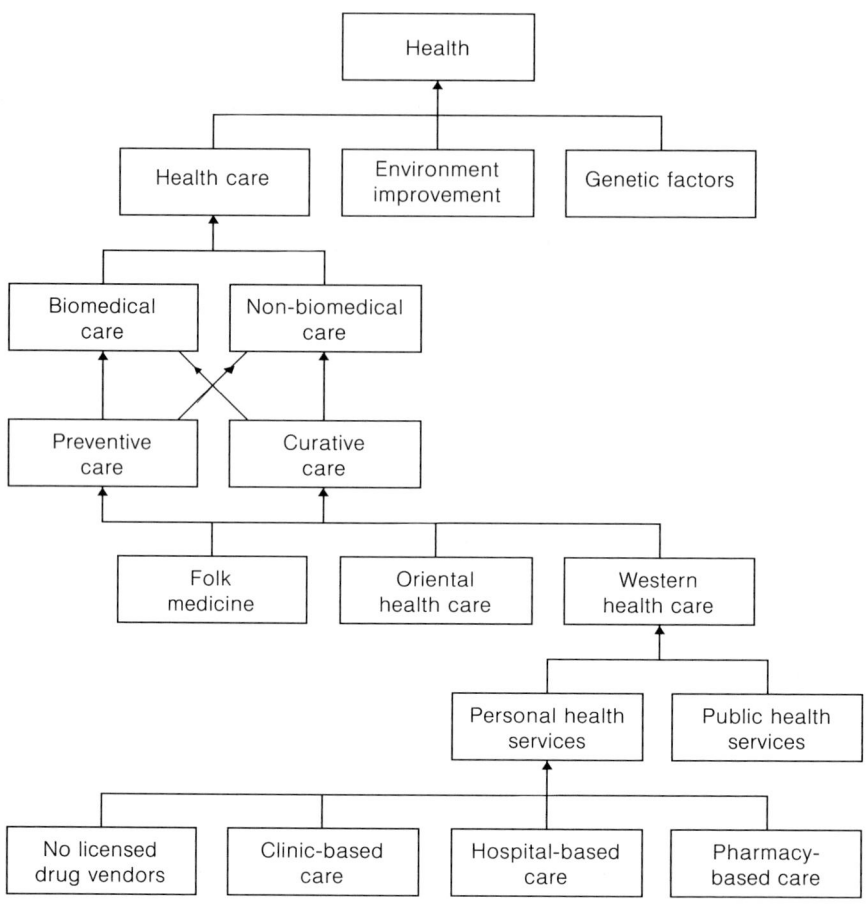

Figure 4. *A schematic view of the allocative process in production of health and utility*

Before any decisions are made about the amount of a nation's limited resources to be spent and the kinds of health technology to be imported, decisions must be made about the allocation of resources between health needs and other needs. Such resource allocation is decided at stage I of the allocative process presented diagrammatically in Figure 4.

At stage I the optimum allocation of resources is achieved when an incremental resource allocated to health brings about an amount of welfare (utility) equal to that produced by an incremental resource allocated to any other "commodity".

Once the total resources to be allocated for the nation's health have been decided, the next stage is the allocation of resources among the various factors that contribute to the improvement of health, which, according to convention, are health-care, environmental and genetic factors (See stage II in Figure 4). Whether an optimum allocation of resources at stage II is achieved should be judged according to the same criterion as at stage I, i.e., the input/output ratios for those three factors have to be equal.

If the input/output ratio for health care is higher than that for improving the environment, resources should be shifted from the provision of health care to the improvement of the environment. In terms of an optimum mix of health technologies, this implies importing more indirect and fewer direct health technologies.

This process of resource allocation can go further. Thus, it can be used in selecting from the technologies that can be used to improve health care the particular kind of technology to be imported. For example, at stage III, if the amount of resources allocated to health manpower (labour) contributes more to the provision of quality health care than does that allocated to health equipment, the technology to be imported should include more, and medical education less, of means of improving health facilities or of equipment. Figure 4 presents the process for health manpower only, but this process and its implications can be applied for each of the three major factors contributing to health.

The economic concept of optimum allocation of resources may be useful for formulating policy strategy for the import of health technology. However, how may this concept be applied?

Its application presents a measurement problem. To ensure that input/output ratios are the same among various factors contributing to health, it must be possible to calculate input and output. Measuring input is not difficult, as the monetary cost of input can represent the amount of resources spent.

The difficulties arise when attempts are made to measure output, i.e. the incremental contribution to health, if we may discuss the allocation process at stage II. There are numerous health status indices. Even if consensus is reached on a composite indicator of health status, how can the amount of contribution made by an input to improving the health indicator be estimated?

The economists' approach is to build a model of production of health. With such a model, the input/output ratio for each factor hypothesized to contribute to the improvement of health may be estimated. Such an estimate is, at best, a rough one. Extreme caution should be exercised, if a model of this kind is to be used.

Another approach applicable is the Delphi method. Experts can get together and "brain-storm". These methods may produce an experts' estimate of the relative size of the contribution to health of each input. Neither method is very reliable. However, the use of this kind of process to achieve an optimum allocation of limited resources among various health technologies to be imported would help developing countries to formulate policy strategies for importing an "appropriate" mix of health technologies.

6. Health Technology Transfer for What Tpes of Health Care?

Health technology transfer has always meant the transfer of Western biomedical technology. However, as many developing countries have relied more on traditional medicine and non-biomedicine than on Western biomedicine it is necessary to examine the problems associated with the transfer of non-Western medicine and of non-biomedicine. In addition, for a given type of medicine, it may also be fruitful to examine the transfer of technology for different categories of health care, such as preventive as compared with curative care, personal as compared with public-health care, and physical as compared with mental health care (Figure 5).

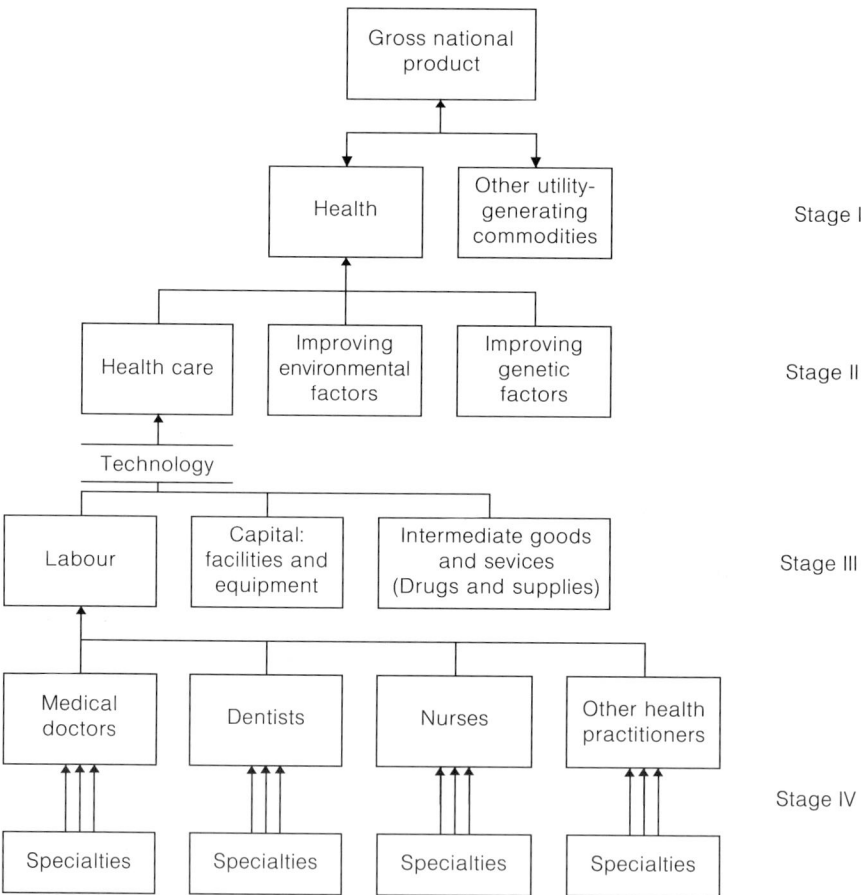

Figure 5. *A schematic view of the allocative process for production of health among different types of health services*

From the perspective of economists the selection of a particular technology for improving the provision of various types of health care can be decided in the same way as that for improving the productivity of various inputs for health or health care.

Policy-makers have to decide which type of health care makes the maximum contribution to improving the nation's health. Then, the technology that improves that type of health care most, for the resources spent, should be imported first.

In other words, once a priority is set among different types of health care, i.e., between Oriental and Western medicine, preventive and curative care, biomedical and non-biomedical care, etc., the technologies to be selected for import should be those that make the maximum contribution to the improvement of the priority type of health care for the resources spent.

This does not imply that only the particular technology that improves the priority type of health care most is to be imported. It implies, rather, a process of deciding on the relative amount of resources to be spent on different technologies, of which each improves a particular type of health care to a varying extent. The objective is the same: to import an optimum mix of technologies among those that improve various types of health care. To repeat, this can be achieved when the input (resource)/output(improvement) ratios are equalized among different technologies for improving various types of health care.

7. Health Technology Exporter-Importer Relationship

The relationship between health-technology exporting and importing countries differs somewhat from that between general-technology exporting and importing countries. In general-technology transfer, the exporting country is willing to transfer only those technologies that will not lessen its competitive advantage in international trade. Indeed, some countries go to great lengths to prevent the leakage of high technology to their potential rivals.

In highly competitive international trade, some countries succeed in maintaining a trade surplus, while others have a chronic trade-deficit. In today's "high-tech" economies, those countries that export more than they import are usually those that possess a comparative technological advantage in manufacturing. Therefore, no one can blame any country that is not willing to share its technological advantage with other countries.

Also, there is keen competition in health-technology transfer among the developed countries. As most developing countries are not expected to become competitors soon after importing health technologies, exporters are tempted to transfer health technology in such ways as to gain advantage over other exporters.

Health-technology transfer can make the recipient country dependent on the exporting country. The packaged health-technology transfer, which includes, *inter alia*, exclusive marketing rights, use of trade marks, and import of service parts, improves the exporting country's competitiveness and increases its profit but it is likely to prolong the reliance of importing countries on foreign technology and slow down the acquisition of their own technological capability.

Tie-in and package sales are common in international trade. However, in health technology transfer, it is widely recognized among policy-makers of both developed and developing countries that it is the responsibility of technology-exporting countries to ensure that transfer improves not only the exporting country's profit but also the importing countries' health and health-technology capabilities. Rather than competing among health-technology exporting countries for a larger share of the international market to gain more profit, these countries should compete in helping the developing and less developed countries gain appropriate health-technology and technology-absorption capabilities.

Since better health contributes to improved human capital, and since improvement in human capital increases labour productivity and improves the economic infrastructure of developing countries, this kind of responsible behaviour in health technology transfer is in the enlightened self-interest of the developed countries. As the importing countries' economies develop, they are likely to become more viable trade partners, to their mutual benefit.

A responsible policy on health technology transfer should also exert a positive influence on the developed country's general trade policy. Those countries that take a moral stand in the export of health technology should take part in formulating policy to prevent the aggressive cigarette-sale campaigns and misleading baby-food-formula marketing by some developed-country companies in developing countries.

The countries that import health technology have some serious responsibilities also. In general trade policy, with limited foreign exchange, developing countries have to make sure that they import mainly those goods and services that contribute to their economic growth. Import of an optimum mix of goods and services, which usually favours the import of investment goods for building a socioeconomic infrastructure over the import of consumer goods, is an important element in determining the success or failure of economic development.

This criterion applies also to the import of health technology by developing countries. It is a responsibility of policy-makers in developing countries to see that the health technology imported is "appropriate". Appropriateness is judged according to the effects that the imported technology would have on the nation's health, its technology absorption capability, equity and socioeconomic development.

For example, for some developing countries the import of highly sophisticated technology might benefit a few, while most people would not have access to basic primary health care. In addition to this equity issue, the imported high technology might not be fully utilized because of lack of ability to use sophisticated equipment. In such circumstances the imported technology makes a minimal contribution to the nation's health and economic development, thus wasting the country's scarce resources.

From an economist's perspective, the developing and less-developed countries should strive for an efficient and equitable health system suitable to their socio-economic and cultural infrastructure, and then within this system formulate sound import policies on health technology, based on economic allocative and production efficiency criteria and the role of human capital in national development.

In summary, health technology transfer can benefit both exporting and importing countries, as a factor in international trade and in its promotion of health and welfare for all. Responsible exporters and importers of health technology should form a sound partnership for their mutual sustained benefit.

8. Conclusion

In conclusion, the transfer of appropriate health technology contributes to the improvement of the recipient country's national development to a greater extent than does the transfer of other technology. This is because transfer of general technology contributes mainly to the economic development of the recipient country by raising its labour productivity through raising the quality of its physical capital. In contrast, health technology transfer contributes to national development mainly by improving human capital. Improvement in human capital not only raises labour productivity but also improves general technological capabilities, which increases both labour and capital productivity.

Recently, economists have shifted emphasis from physical to human capital as the main contributor to building socioeconomic infrastructure and to accelerating national development. It has been estimated that from 40 to 60% of recent increase in gross national product of many developed countries has been made by investment in human capital in the form of education and health.

Sustained improvement in human capital contributes to human welfare by improving efficiency of both production and consumption. This means that healthy and more educated people both benefit more from, and contribute more to, rising living standards.

By improving human capital, the transfer of appropriate health technology contributes also to the recipient country's capacity to absorb technology and to accelerate development. This has cumulative effects, as improved technological capabilities lead to further technological progress and to the development of the recipient country's own technological basis.

Once a nation succeeds in building a "critical mass" of human capital of high quality, it sets in motion a positive circle. The improved human capital in greater quantity leads to more investment in human and physical capital and to further technological progress and economic growth. These in turn have cumulative effects on investment in physical and human capital, enabling a developing country to reach the so-called "take-off" point.

103

For the transfer of health technology to be able to contribute significantly to the ability of developing countries to reach the take-off point, several pre-conditions have to be met. These are: socioeconomic and cultural infrastructure, a favourable political environment, and an essential minimum basis of capacity to absorb technology.

Even with these conditions, a mutually beneficial and sustainable partnership has to be built between the exporter and the importer of health technology. The exporting country must have a genuine interest in improving the health and the human capital of the importing country. The importing or recipient country has to have a sound policy in prioritizing investment in various programmes and in various types of health technology imports. The transfer of appropriate health technology on the basis of a sound donor-recipient partnership can make a significant contribution to the attainment of WHO's goal of health for all by the year 2000.

HEALTH TECHNOLOGY TRANSFER: THE PERSPECTIVE OF HEALTH MINISTRIES OF DEVELOPING COUNTRIES

S.D.M. Fernando*

1. Historical background—the need for reorientation of health systems

As late as four decades ago, the majority of countries classified as "developing countries" were parts of Western colonial empires and their health systems were modelled essentially on those of the colonial powers. The colonial era was one of great scientific and technological achievement in England and the other European colonial countries. In such a technology-oriented framework the health systems that developed in the West were essentially hospital-based, with priority accorded to curative care. At the same time the need to control epidemics resulted in some growth also of public health and community medicine. In the colonies too, the health systems were heavily biased towards hospital and curative services, and very inadequate provision was made for prevention and health promotion. This was essentially the position at the end of World War II, in the mid-'forties. Therefore as former colonies in Asia, Africa and the Americas gained their independence in the late 'forties and in the 'fifties and 'sixties, ministries of health in the newly independent countries inherited health systems designed primarily to provide curative care, and that only for the more economically advanced segments of their populations.

The advent of antibiotics, which resulted in what were perceived as "miracle cures" for such dreaded diseases as typhoid fever, pneumonia, venereal diseases, malaria and diphtheria, increased further the popularity of hospitals, and in the early years after independence health ministries of the developing countries, as the former colonies were labelled, allocated resources primarily for the expansion of their hospital networks. This included the establishment of medical and nursing schools, which were carbon copies of their Western counterparts. It soon became clear, however, that though hospital-based health systems had a marked impact on mortality it continued to remain high among the more disadvantaged and vulnerable groups of society, especially mothers and children.

Consequently, the developing countries realized that health systems similar to those of the developed world were not suitable means for tackling their health problems. Their health ministries saw that the emphasis in health system development had to be changed from curative to promotive and preventive health care. Thus by the late 'fifties and

* Director of Health Services, Ministry of Health and Women's Affairs, Colombo, Sri Lanka.

early 'sixties they had recognized that the development of health infra-structure had to be reoriented, in regard to both the functioning of physical facilities and the training of health manpower, including doctors and nurses.

The early efforts at reorientation to control their pressing health problems, such as smallpox, malaria and venereal diseases, resulted in the establishment of disease-control programmes that functioned as vertical programmes. These had varying degrees of success, but brought no obvious reduction of the burden of disease or improvement in quality of life. Therefore in the late 'sixties and early 'seventies, health ministries of developing countries began to favour and adopt the "basic health services" approach, which culminated in the mid 'seventies in integration becoming the focus of policy.

At the same time it became clear that reorientation of health systems to meet the needs of all the people could not be separated from development in general, concerned with, for example, housing, water supply, sanitation, food supply and nutrition, road networks, transport and communication systems. These had to be viewed in relation to the development of health systems, with emphasis on promotive and pre-ventive health.

2. Change in perspective: the goal of health for all

The adoption of the goal of health for all by the year 2000 by the World Health Assembly in 1977, and the Alma-Ata Declaration on primary health care, in 1978, provided the basis and impetus for change that ministries of health in developing countries had sought in order to adjust their health systems so as to meet the health needs of all their people.

The primary-health-care concept also indicated the way in which resources should be redistributed to obtain maximum results, by provid-ing health care which would be accessible, affordable and of high quality, and technologically and scientifically sound. Primary health care also had a definite political dimension welcomed by policy-makers in developing countries, since it emphasized equity and social justice in the provision of health care. The other important facets of the primary-health-care approach are: focus on prevention, appropriate technology, community involvement and intersectoral cooperation.

Therefore in the decade of the 'eighties, health ministries in the developing countries changed their approach to the provision of care from an essentially hospital-based system to one of comprehensive health care focusing on health promotion and prevention of disease, while maintaining high standards of curative care provided at different levels of referral. National strategies based on this new approach were imple-mented. The active involvement of communities and health-related sectors became integral to the reorientation that took place within the health system. The focus shifted from the treatment of individuals to the care of families and communities.

It is also important to remember that, while reordering priorities to meet the challenge of health for all, the ministries of health of the developing countries have continued to provide good-quality curative care with far fewer resources than are available in the developed world. Indeed, it is doubtful whether the developed countries could provide such care to their people under the conditions prevailing in developing countries, such as shortage of trained medical and nursing personnel, limited infrastructure and deficient logistics. To take a simple example, during an operating session in a developing-country hospital 12 operations will be completed, compared with only four in a developed country. The point being emphasized is that what the developing countries have achieved with the resources at their disposal could not perhaps have been achieved in the developed countries, with their focus still on care of individual patients in hospital-centred systems of health care, had they been faced with the problems of the developing countries.

3. Reorientation of health systems for primary health care

With the changed perspective of the ministries of health in the developing countries after the Alma-Ata Conference, several significant adjustments were made in their health systems. Managerial processes and mechanisms were reoriented to implement effectively the new strategies. This included the restructuring and reorganization of ministries of health. Reorganization was aimed primarily at improving the coordination of curative and preventive services, and at integrating "vertical" health programmes into the general health services. Greater attention was given to clarifying functions of staff at different levels of the health system, and to decentralizing authority. Legislation was enacted to support the policies of reorientation. The emphasis on training of health manpower changed to meet the needs of the new direction in the delivery of health care. As the infrastructure expanded and more physical facilities were established at primary care level, community health workers were trained to work in these new facilities. Team-work and team-training were emphasized in the training of primary-health-care workers. Activities to reorient medical education for primary health care also commenced. Reorientation of the health system for primary health care highlighted the need to deal with behavioural issues, in the interaction of health workers with communities and with other, health-related sectors. As the management of health services required a familiarity with social issues, which had not been part of the traditional functions of medical and other health workers, programmes were initiated for training health managers at all levels, especially the middle-level management grades. To address problems associated with reorientation the discipline of health systems research and development began to receive more attention. Together with the reorientation of health manpower training, mechanisms to institutionalize health systems research were also initiated in many developing countries.

Therefore in the ten years following the Alma-Ata Conference and Declaration, the views of the ministries of health of the developing countries on the direction of health system development underwent radical change. In March 1988, WHO convened a meeting at Riga,

USSR, to determine the extent to which the new approaches, especially in developing countries, had improved health status and quality of life.

4. Review of achievements

The meeting at Riga, which was held at roughly the midpoint between the Alma-Ata Conference and the year 2000, concluded that most countries had made considerable gains in increasing the equity and effectiveness of health services and in improving the health and well-being of their populations. Considerable improvement had taken place in coverage, effectiveness and equality of programmes. For example:

- Many countries had based their national health policies on the concepts of health for all, emphasizing health promotion, including improvement in life-styles, and decentralizing initiatives to districts, cities and local communities.
- Immunization rates had increased from about 5% of children in developing countries in 1970 to more than 50% in the late 1980s.
- Infant, under-five and maternal mortality had decreased remarkably: in many countries the under-five mortality rates had decreased by more than 50% since 1950.

This showed that the change in the approaches of health ministries had indeed resulted in many creditable achievements. However, the Riga meeting noted that the gains, though widespread, were not uniform either between or within countries. A number of least developed countries had made only limited progress; their infant, young-child and maternal mortality rates and related morbidities remained unacceptably high. Also, health problems were increasing in large urban populations of developing countries.

The meeting highlighted the fact that in many developing countries the standards of health of some segments of the population were still far below what would be acceptable. They still lacked adequate income, nutrition, education and sanitation, safe drinking water and comprehensive health care. To mitigate these problems and continue to build upon the successes already achieved, the Riga meeting suggested ten action areas, all of which are relevant to health ministries in developing countries.

They are:

(1) Maintaining health for all as a permanent goal of all nations up to and beyond the year 2000.

(2) Renewing and strengthening strategies for health for all.

(3) Intensifying social and political action for health.

(4) Developing and mobilizing leadership for health for all.

(5) Empowering people.

(6) Making intersectoral collaboration a force for health for all.

(7) Strengthening district health systems based on primary health care.

(8) Planning, preparing and supporting health personnel for health for all.

(9) Ensuring the development and rational use of science and appropriate technology.

(10) Overcoming problems that continue to resist solutions.

5. Proposals for future action

There is no doubt that the health ministries of developing countries have been proceeding along the right path in their policies and plans of action for achieving health for all. What is required now is to continue on this path, making further adjustments in the health system, based on the recommendations of the Riga meeting. A few important activities for which health ministries could provide leadership are given below:

(a) To intensify community involvement, which is both a technical and a social necessity. Health ministries should pay greater attention to this factor. It should not be forgotten that empowering the people is integral to community involvement.

(b) To place strong emphasis on the development of leaders at community, district and national levels, since there is a clear need for leadership in health and other sectors at all levels.

(c) Health ministries should make greater and more concerted efforts to make intersectoral action a potent force in their strategies. The approach for the future should be to promote health through public policies, emphasizing that health development is integral to all socio-economic development, and therefore improves quality of life as well as health status.

(d) The district health system should be further strengthened, because the district is well suited to overcoming problems of health services in relation to community development.

(e) With regard to the development of human resources for health, three aspects are important: the need for integrated health systems and manpower development; the need to strengthen the preparation of health personnel as regards relevance to health needs and demands; and the need to counter the sense of severe demoralization of health personnel in many field settings.

Continuing political commitment of the highest order is vital if the efforts of the health ministries are to succeed. Yet political commitment by itself has limitations, without the resources for translating commitment into action. To obtain such resources health ministries must challenge current international development thought, which discounts investment in health and other social sectors in favour of economic improvement only.

Efforts should be undertaken to enhance the international climate for development support. This should include policies that focus on social equity rather than economic considerations alone, and that recognize the long-term nature of social development and promote wider understanding and acceptance of the development process, including respect for the people who are involved in its implementation. The success of the plans of health ministries depends to a great extent on adequate financing of health systems.

THE ROLE OF THE THIRD-WORLD UNIVERSITY IN BRIDGING THE TRANSFER OF TECHNOLOGY FROM THE FIRST TO THE THIRD WORLD

J.H. Bryant, P.C. Erwin and A.A. Farrukhi*

Introduction

The problems of technology transfer are pervasive in the Third World. True dilemmas occur:

— there are opportunities to advance national capabilities by absorbing recently developed technologies, but to do so requires excessive consumption of resources that are badly needed to meet basic needs.

Instances of inadvertent or even foolish wastage abound:

— the new machine is highly desirable but complex to set up and maintain, and sits in its shipping container, unused and deteriorating.

Such dilemmas and wastage are to be seen on every side in the health field, and there the cost in human terms is often very great:

— rising costs of 21st century technology bloat the budgets of urban hospitals, while rural communities live in 15th century conditions without effective health services;
— technologies are available that are relevant to widespread problems and affordable but that are not being applied, because the problems are overlooked or the knowledge to use the technology is not locally available, or the local health services are stagnant, and the ill remain ill, or die.

The Bridging Function of the Third-World University in Technology Transfer
In the face of such problems, the Third-World university has a special role to play. It stands astride the gap between First-World and Third-World technologies.

On the one side are deep poverty, widespread and barely-checked diseases, sparseness and fragility of health services, social and political uncertainty, and the thinly developed base of science and educational systems of the Third World.

* Department of Community Health Sciences, Aga Khan University, Karachi, Pakistan.

On the other side are rapid advances in science and technology in multiple fields, developed in the laboratories and field settings of universities, governmental research programmes and industry, with rapid communication and diffusion of ideas, materials and products, adjusting to cost constraints, capitalizing on economic demand, and often hungry for Third-World markets.

A Third-World university has open access to both sides. The question is: can the university help to bridge the gap, and bring the one to assist the other in constructive ways, or will it use indiscriminately its access to First World technology and thereby become part of the problem?

The Aga Khan University in Karachi, Pakistan has been grappling with these dilemmas and challenges, and believes that the Third-World university has a special role to play in balancing technology transfer with the needs and dynamics of Third World development.

The key issue is the bridging function:

Done carefully, there can be sharing of ideas, concepts, technologies, sensitivities, methods, materials, cultural values and people;

Done carelessly, there can be distorted interpretations of need, blind transfers of unneeded technologies, ruinous financial burdens, and mindless disregard of cultural values. In reality, there will be some of both. But where will the balance be?

A natural ally of the Third-World university is the First-World university, but there are gaps in this alliance as well:

In First-World universities, there are numerous personnel and predictable career paths, libraries, equipment, stable institutions, attractive monetary packages, and rich networks of academic communications and support;

In Third-World universities, too often there are understaffed institutions and uncertain career paths, libraries with half-empty and dusty shelves, poorly maintained equipment, unstable institutions and lean networks of academic communication.

However, while coping with its own deficiencies, the Third-World university can use its alliances with First-World universities in grappling with the problem of technology transfer.

Linking University Action with National Health Policies
Pakistan presents a paradigm of health policy in the making. With a newly elected government, a new National Health Policy is being formulated, which gives close attention to strengthening health services, with equity as a prime objective. The Aga Khan University is a partner with government and others in helping to implement the Policy. One step is to assist in the formulation of a research agenda for the National Health Policy, which will culminate in 1990 in a National Workshop on Policy-Related Health Research[3].

Implementation of the Policy calls for addressing deep deficiencies in existing systems. *To a large extent the deficiencies are not in the development of new technologies but in the application of known technolo-*

111

gies, many of them managerial. Here, the development process is critical: there can be no implementation of systems copied and imported from abroad. Prototypes must be developed locally, adjusted according to local conditions and customs, used for staging widespread expansion, in hopes of reaching equity through revitalized health services.

An interesting and important step is the transfer of knowledge and technology developed in local prototypes to the governmental systems required for widespread diffusion—that is, *transfer within the country.* The government may not have the immediate capacity to absorb the prototype, and attention has to be given to strengthening its capacity so that the chain of events from technology development to testing to implementation is not broken.

In underdeveloped societies, the chain from technology development to application is often fragile and easily broken. Understanding, monitoring and strengthening it are as important as the technology itself.

Methods of Assessing Technology for Third World Application
Certain methods are particularly appropriate for assessing the usefulness of technologies in Third World settings, where a prime determinant of appropriateness of technology is the extent to which it supports or detracts from resources that should be reserved for poor and remote populations. Two methods that can be used for this purpose are epidemiology and cost-effectiveness analysis.

> Epidemiology can help to determine whether there is a positive relation between a given intervention and a desired outcome: did the administration of vitamin A reduce infant mortality?
>
> Cost-effectiveness analysis can help determine the cost of the intervention in relation to the effect: if proven effective, would the administration of vitamin A to target populations be affordable?

By applying these methods of analysis to populations, the problem of intensive care for a few versus the needs of many can be addressed. The following example serves to highlight these issues:

In its commitment to equity the Department of Community Health Sciences of the Aga Khan University has established primary-health-care (PHC) field sites in several *katchi abadis* (squatter settlements) of Karachi. In these poor and crowded populations the use of appropriate technology is most critical: resources are precariously thin and the needs are very great.

The Department translates this principle of care according to need by first providing a floor of health services to all in a defined catchment area, then by epidemiological methods identifying those at greatest risk and focusing on them additional resources. Two examples of these relatively-low-technology health services are:

> Immunizations—Community health workers (CHWs) in their daily home visits encourage mothers to bring their children to the health centre for immunization. In addition, immunization services have been mobilized to permit families reluctant (or unable) to come to the centre to have access to these services essentially outside their doors.

Growth monitoring—a "simple" tool that allows us to identify families with malnourished children, which can receive concentrated attention from community health workers.

While the technology of epidemiology can be useful in the design of health services, it can also be used to assess information on utilization of these low-technology services. A recently completed study at the University serves as an example. Our management information system, based on data collected by CHWs, showed that despite the activities of the PHC systems the catchment areas continued to suffer from high child-mortality. As a first step in attempting to answer the question—Why?—and again, by epidemiological methods, we compared families that had experienced a recent child death with families that had never experienced a child death. These "case" and "control" families had been similarly exposed to contaminated environments and were of similar sociocultural background, yet differed in their experience with child deaths (and, thus, with child health).

Of the numerous socioeconomic, demographic and health characteristics compared, only three factors were consistently (i.e., as shown by various analytical methods) significantly different between case and control families: occupation of fathers, family nutrition status, and immunization status.

Fathers' occupations were characterized by the regularity (as opposed to the amount) of income: a steady, regular source of income (monthly wages) compared with an erratic one (daily wages). Families without child deaths were almost four times as likely to have had a steady source of income than were families that had experienced a recent child death. It is possible that stability of income affects the stability of the household, in relation to care of children.

Immunization status and nutritional status of families were based on the status of the children below the age of five years in those families. Information on family immunization and nutrition originated from CHWs' records: these data thus follow the use or implementation of services provided on the basis of care according to need (epidemiologically determined). Yet, the study results may have implications that go beyond the usual interpretation of risk factors. For example, diseases preventable by immunization were not major causes of childhood mortality in these populations; therefore, it is possible that immunization as a specific instance of health-related behaviour of families is an indicator of general behaviour that contributes to the health of their children. Nutritional status also may be seen as an indicator of healthy child-care practices; it may be possible to monitor changes in child-care behaviour by tracking immunization and nutrition levels over time. We believe this study will help us in identifying high-risk households and will provide the impetus for looking more closely at what those "healthy child-care practices" are[4].

Thus one health technology—epidemiology—can be used not only to guide us in the appropriate use of other health technologies—growth monitoring and immunization—but also to help us in understanding the information generated by the use of those other health technologies.

Cost-effectiveness studies could follow epidemiological studies, by measuring the costs of these technologies against their impact.

Support Systems for Technology Transfer: A Future View
Too often in the transfer of technology, a key missing link is a support system for technology use. This support may come in many forms, including manpower (trained technicians), spare parts and information systems. What is also frequently not realized is that these support systems themselves may be examples of technology transfer. The following scenario illustrates this:

The year is 1992:
A call comes to the University from the Ministry of Health with a question:
Negotiation has been under way between government and industry—to buy lithotripters (1991 model, low cost, high efficiency!) for district hospitals in arid areas with high incidence of renal stones.
Under the National Health Care Technology Policy, established in 1991, the government established a Standing Committee with guidelines that called for review of large expenditure on Health Care Technology.
The capital investment of this proposal exceeds the established threshold and the Ministry called the University, which had agreed to maintain WHO's Advisory Data Base on Health Care Technology.
The University expert on radiological systems was called and after brief reflection turned to the library. He sat at the CDROM reader, turned on the attached IBM-compatible PC, and inserted the compact disc entitled:
WHO Health Care Technology Data Base References, Abstracts, Advisory Options Produced by WHO Task Force on Technology Transfer
July—December 1991... Update.
Within five minutes, the relevant materials were on the screen:
Technology Assessment—Lithotripter Applications in Third World Countries.
32 References with abstracts were available.
A key reference was on cost-effectiveness in least developed countries.
The back-up articles were also contained on the disc, and the key article was called up and printed.
The radiologist read the paper and decided it contained the scientific basis for an opinion on the lithotripter question.
He dictated his opinion, and faxed to the Ministry of Health the relevant materials from the Data Base, the key article and his own opinion.
Elapsed time: one hour.

Science fiction? Of course not. CDROM (compact disc, read only memory) technology is already widely available, and the equipment and discs are no more costly than inexpensive computer components. We now have that technology in our departmental library in Pakistan, with access to the entire Index Medicus on a single disc.

Two steps are necessary to bring this story to reality. The first is for WHO to establish a task force on technology transfer, which would develop the technology-assessment data-bases of the kind referred to. The second is for countries to establish national health care technology policies, and mechanisms for relating the policies to uses of the data-bases. In Pakistan, for example, where there is a new, strongly equity-oriented, national health policy, a concerned approach to technology transfer is already apparent.

Ethical Implications of Technology Transfer
Ethical questions abound in the transfer of technology, with special implications for Third World countries[5,6], including at least the following areas of concern:

- Advances in biomedical technology precipitate new ethical dilemmas world-wide, and the movement of technology from First to Third World settings carries with it the same ethical dilemmas.
- Possibly the questions that present the most difficult choices for Third World countries with very high mortality and morbidity rates have to do with balancing the moral weight of expending resources on life-sustaining treatment for vulnerable individuals against the moral weight of protecting resources committed to the needs of larger populations. For example, intensive neonatal-care units—high-tech, high-cost facilities—can save the lives of small numbers of desperately ill infants, with a trade-off against very high infant-mortality rates: 400,000 infant deaths a year in a country of 100 million inhabitants. The difficult choices to be made in trying to balance equity and scarcity require consideration of special decision criteria in very poor countries.
- Ethical questions about technology arise in Third-World settings, to be recognized locally and dealt with in local terms.
- Ethical questions must be resolved according to the values of each society, and, although many societal values are universal in their form and meaning, some are culture-specific, and such specificity must be understood and respected.
- Third-World countries often do not have mechanisms for dealing with decisions on ethical problems, and there is a need to build a capacity and even decision-making structures for dealing with such ethical questions.

The Third-World university, in its bridging role, is especially well placed to deal with the difficult choices that must be made in the application of ethical principles to technology transfer in local settings.

Concluding Reflections

Thus, the Third-World university that would serve the bridging function of monitoring, facilitating and adapting technology transfers to Third-World settings must have both deep roots in Third-World settings and firm connections with First-World technological advances. Both ends of the bridge must be carefully built. Ultimately it is judgment based on understanding of the two sides which will advance the chances of balanced and equity-oriented Third-World development.

References

[1] Bryant, J.H. The Role of the University in Health Manpower Development in a Developing Country. In: *Proceedings of the First Convocation of the Aga Khan University,* Karachi, Pakistan, 1990. In preparation.

[2] National Health Policy of Pakistan. Government of Pakistan, 1990.

[3] Research Agenda of the National Health Policy of Pakistan, 1990. In preparation.

[4] Erwin, P.C., Smith, K., Panjwani, S. and Khan, K.S., Child Mortality in the Squatter Settlements of Karachi, Pakistan, 1989.

[5] *Health Policy. Ethics and Human Values—An International Dialogue.* Highlights of the Athens Conference. Edited by John H. Bryant and Zbigniew Bankowski. CIOMS, Geneva, 1985.

[6] *Health Policy, Ethics, and Human Values—European and North American Perspectives.* Edited by Zbigniew Bankowski and John H. Bryant. CIOMS, Geneva, 1988.

HEALTH TECHNOLOGY TRANSFER: INFRASTRUCTURAL AND MANPOWER NEEDS OF DEVELOPING COUNTRIES

A. Mallouppas*

1. The Problem

At present in developing countries there is an inability to provide efficient, effective, safe and affordable health care at all levels, owing mainly to the lack of technical know-how, tradition and infrastructure of national Health Care Technical Services (HCTS). The problem is exacerbated by the limited availability of foreign currency and the influx of high technology at all levels and types of equipment. The general economic and logistic support that the health sector needs from other sectors of the national system, such as roads and telecommunications, is largely wanting, and inefficient operation of customs procedures and of inter-sector coordination, poor collaboration and weak management worsen an already adverse situation.

2. Major Consequences of Present Situation

There is therefore an appreciable wastage of limited national resources, as the following table shows.

Cause	Estimated Waste
– Purchase of sophisticated equipment, which is under-used or never used, owing to lack of operating and maintenance staff and medical expertise to support and use it	20%–40% of equipment
– Limitation of the useful life-time of equipment due to inexperience of operators and lack of servicing	Reduced by 30%–80%
– Additional purchase of accessories, extras, specialized spare parts and testing equipment and building modifications, initially unforeseen owing to lack of expertise in choosing appropriate systems in the first place	10%–30% of value of equipment
– Lack of standardization resulting in increased costs of spare parts and extra work-load on the limited competent staff	30%–50% extra spare-parts costs

---

* Head WHO Collaborating Centre for Training and Research on Maintenance and Repair of Health Care Equipment, Higher Technical Institute, Nicosia, Cyprus.

– Excessive down-time of equipment, i.e. time they remain inoperative, owing to lack of spare parts, inexperience in repair and lack of preventive maintenance	25%–50% of equipment
– Lack of liquidity in foreign exchange reserves, which forces countries to accept unfavourable purchasing contracts	10%–30% extra purchasing costs of equipment and spares

3. Identification of the Major Obstacles Facing the Health Sector

It is obvious that the obstacles that impede the health sector can be overcome only if other national sectors also improve, such as roads and logistic support, telecommunications, and management and coordination within the government service.

The four major obstacles in developing countries are:

- lack of organizational policy;
- ineffective health care technical service (HCTS);
- inadequate manpower development and training; and
- insufficient information support.

3.1. Lack of organizational policy

At present inadequate awareness of the magnitude and complexity of an adequate system of health-care technical services, and the limited expertise of policy-makers, planners and managers, prevent the necessary policy formulation, planning development, securing of funding and identification of all aspects that must be considered in defining effective policies on the management of health-care equipment.

A complicated cycle of events must be taken into account in planning for meeting national health needs, based on medical necessity. At the stage of policy formulation, decision-making should involve in a collective team approach all the parties concerned with the management of equipment; decisions should not be made by individuals or separate services.

Once the health needs have been identified, the necessary interventions must be taken into account. These include types of equipment, physical facilities, funding requirements, logistic support, and local market support, particularly in spare parts and technical information. Equipment procurement involves the determination and quantification of general technical specifications, spare-parts needs, personnel training (both user and service staff), and service-workshop facilities in calibration and testing of equipment. This must be done and the facilities made available at or before the installation of the equipment.

3.2. Ineffective Health Care Technical Service (HCTS)

The inadequacies in infrastructure (human resources and physical facilities), organizational capability, expertise, training, incentives and career structure, funding and collaboration with other sectors are such that they render the HCTS ineffective and inefficient.

To produce the expected results the HCTS must be given the necessary inputs.

Committed government policy is a prerequisite for an adequate budget, planning programmes, spare parts, physical facilities, staff posts, career structure, etc. Having the required inputs is not enough to produce the desirable results, which are proper selection, specification and procurement of equipment, planning, inventory control, routine preventive maintenance, repairs and training of staff (user and service). Since many developing countries have no tradition or background in the servicing of equipment, their staff are unable to deliver quickly the expected results. Today's fast-changing electronics technology is not making matters easier.

The HCTS at central and provincial level should be able to carry out the following tasks:

- Identification of health needs
- Programming and planning of health interventions
- Policy, infrastructure and organization of HCTS
- Identification of needs in manpower, facilities, supplies, etc.
- Recruitment, promotion and assessment of staff
- Identification of equipment needs
- Financing policies for purchases and replacements
- Inventory control and updating
- Quality and safety control of equipment
- Control of imported equipment, sources and evaluation
- Equipment selection, specification, tendering, procurement
- Identification of trainng and retraining needs of users and technical staff
- Policy on spare parts and technical documentation
- Identification and planning of physical facilities and needs
- Requirements in routine maintenance, calibration and testing facilities
- Evaluation of private-sector support
- Collaboration with other services and organizations

Thus, short-term and long-term programmes of manpower development and strengthening of service workshops should be designed and implemented to enable the HCTS to perform its tasks.

The main indicators of maintenance effectiveness of the HCTS are:

- Availability of service workshops at all levels (fully staffed and equipped with necessary transport support)
- Inventory at central, provincial and hospital levels
- Planned preventive maintenance programmes at all levels with necessary monitoring systems
- Adequate supply of common spare parts
- Full technical library at each workshop
- Selection of equipment according to health needs and by means of a team approach

119

- Adequate career structure and staff posts
- Trained and experienced personnel
- Liaison with local and international market
- Availability of local training within national capabilities and needs
- Effective reporting system for repairs
- Low down-time of equipment
- Annual statistics relating to efficiency and effectiveness of service and equipment utilization

3.3. Inadequate development and training of manpower

The present lack of career structures, low levels of salaries, and inadequacy of staff development and training for both user and service personnel at all levels of the health sector, including technical managers, inhibit staff members from fulfilling their responsibilities adequately.

Manpower development should cover all levels of the service, i.e. central, provincial, district and rural. The latter two should be provided for by National Training Centres. These are still not widely found in developing countries; their establishment should be actively promoted.

National-level training programmes should:

- initially provide for Artisan and Polyvalent (General) Technician level (Annex I);
- be within national capabilities and needs, commencing if necessary with expatriate assistance.

National Training Centres should be situated in established technical institutions at central and, for very large countries, provincial levels. However, they should be very closely linked to HCTS Central Maintenance Workshops situated in large general hspitals. In this way hospital (on-the-job) training could be carried out in a large hospital environment, where students would be exposed to a large variety of problems.

International (regional or interregional) training is still required for higher-level Specialized Technician, Assistant Engineer and Engineer training. Such centres exist already in some regions. A comprehensive international training programme would need the coordinating support of WHO for ensuring the necessary transfer of expertise and training materials and establishing higher-level training, particularly for Engineer or Assistant Engineer, which is essential and at present cannot be undertaken at national level.

3.4. Insufficient information support

Today's rapid technological changes call for the availability of adequate and up-dated technical information for user, service and planning personnel. Of particular importance is information related to health-care equipment installation and commissioning, operating practices, safety standards, quality control, servicing, repairs, technical library and data, and information about manufacturers and equipment.

Trainers as well as staff of the Health Care Technical Service need to have up-to-date information about equipment in order to use it, suitably modified and implemented, for national needs. It would thus be highly

120

appropriate for WHO to act as a coordinator and distributor of information on computer data-banks, equipment codes, practices, safety and hazard notices, plant preventive maintenance procedures, etc. To achieve this objective national information systems need to be set up, capable of handling, adapting and assimilating such information and then ensuring that it is suitably implemented by the appropriate departments. Their incorporation in a National Training Centre could result in a National Training and Information Centre or in several such centres, whose staff would provide both training and information support. The equipment needed for national information systems includes a personal-computer system and a heavy-duty photocopier, for storing information and distributing it to the various health sectors and the Health Care Technical Service, as well as fax, telex, printing, packaging and mailing facilities.

To realize needs arising from the use of high technology, to implement effective and efficient Health Care Technical Services, and to provide adequate information transfer and support, a high calibre of trained and experienced staff is necessary. The required courses must therefore be organized at international level to make such training available to staff from developing countries.

4. Proposed Strategy and Approach

To improve the present situation, and because of its interdependent and interactive nature, there is a need to strengthen cooperation between Health Care Technical Services and the local market, financial support and management, medical stores, transport and logistic support systems, medical and para-medical personnel, and customs procedures.

To address the four major obstacles mentioned earlier it is necessary to:

- improve awareness, policy formulation, planning development and implementation;
- strengthen the effectiveness and efficiency of Health Care Technical Services and the standard of service offered;
- promote mechanisms to improve working and career conditions and offer adequate training to *all* staff at *all* levels of the health sector;
- identify and implement the means of collecting, collating, assessing, disseminating and updating technical information.

5. Conclusions

The above suggestions are aimed at improving the management, maintenance and repair of health-care equipment. This is essential if the health-care benefits of technology are to be fully applied to the improvement of health-care delivery in developing countries.

6. Recommendations

To achieve the above, the following are necessary:

- Awareness seminars on policy formulation and planning development for technical managers and engineers of Health Care Technical Services;
- The strengthening or establishment of service workshops at central, provincial and district hospitals, with adequate staff, facilities and equipment capable of offering service-support to rural and urban health units in their areas;
- The strengthening or establishment of national training centres to provide initially for the training of technicians for basic medical equipment, for national needs and within national capabilities;
- The establishment of national information systems, using data-banks capable of collecting, collating and disseminating technical information to interested parties within the health sector;
- The establishment of national focal points to liaise with international agencies and manufacturers on matters concerning training, information transfer and bilateral agreements, equipment information and data;
- The establishment of a standing policy-and-planning committee comprising members representing *all* interested parties (medical, technical and user staff, finance, etc.) to oversee equipment policy and identify health needs;
- The strengthening of regional and interregional training centres to enable them to offer training not available or envisaged in the near future at national level.

ANNEX I

Example of outline syllabus for a polyvalent technician course

Syllabus: Subject Matter

1. **English**
   Includes Oral and Reading Skills, Grammar, Vocabulary of Technical English, Letter and Report Writing.

2. **Mathematics**
   Includes Computation, Logarithms, Trigonometry, Basic algebraic equations, Graphical representation.

3. **Technical Drawing**
   Includes use of technical drawing instruments, Elementary constructions, Pictorial projection, Sections, Electrical drawing, Visualization.

4. **Workshops**
   Includes Electrical installations, theory and practice of wiring (domestic and industrial), selection of cables, lighting circuits, earthing systems, types of lamps. Principles and practice of: Arc welding, Gas welding, Sheet metal, Plumbing. Bench fitting: Use of files, hacksaw, chisels, drills and drilling. Threads, piping systems, workshop maintenance.

5. **Electronics and Electrotechnics**
   Includes Electrical measurements, DC and AC circuits, Electrical components, Transformers, AC and DC motors, Semi-conductors, Power supplies, Amplifiers, Applications of transistors, DIACS and TRIACS.

6. **Mechanical Services** (Hospital Plant)
   Includes Heating and Hot Water Services, Refrigeration, Ventilation and Air conditioning, lubricants, stand-by generators, test vehicles repair and servicing.

7. **Medical Equipment**
   Includes principles, operation and simple repairs and maintenance of the following equipment: Blood-pressure meters, stethoscopes, water baths, microscopes, autoclaves, sterilizers, trolleys, basic mechanical medical equipment, suction machines, centrifuges, theatre light, lamps, etc.

8. **Hospital Field Work**
   Field work under supervision in hospital workshops, involving simple repairs and maintenance.

Duration: One year

Entrance Requirements: Candidates for the course should be graduates of a secondary technical school and preferably have some practical experience in a hospital workshop or technical service. Also a basic command of the English language would be an advantage.

FACILITATORS OF TRANSFER

THE PERSPECTIVE OF INTERNATIONAL ORGANIZATIONS IN HEALTH TECHNOLOGY TRANSFER

M. Abdelmoumène*

So much has been said and written about technology transfer that I believe it is high time for us in WHO to attempt a leap forward. Although I do not believe in magic recipes, I do believe in scientific research and in brain power. The problems that confront us in world health are so immense, and our resources and knowledge for coping with them so insufficient, that we need an urgent programme of action to try to reduce the disparity.

The picture of inequality in health technology is dominated by the tragic burden of morbidity and mortality borne by countries of the Third World. Although some kind of industrial parity between a wealthy region of the globe and a poor one can be quickly achieved, perhaps by transferring turnkey operations, the same cannot be said of health parity. The toll of disease and poverty in the South is the result of fundamental societal and economic processes, of an evolutionary nature, which are not amenable to "quick-fix" methods.

The fact that more than four-fifths of the world's output is produced by the North, and that most of the South cannot spend more than 0.2% of its gross national product on research and development has been abundantly documented. It is of particular relevance that disparities between the North and the South, per capita, could range in magnitude between a hundred and a thousand times, depending on the particular geographical region or population subgroup under consideration.

The spectacular pace of scientific and technological advance in post-industrial societies underlines the inability of the Third World to afford to reshape the frontiers of knowledge. Yet, the cliché about a widening gap has to be qualified: for example, the production rates of scientists and engineers in the North and in the South are converging rapidly.

Programmes for development have been prescribed in many forums, including WHO. Most people will agree that the following outline is based on reasonable principles.

Firstly, that political will should be fostered and express itself by the establishment of appropriate coordinating and promotional mechanisms.

Secondly, that national policies on health technology should be formulated with clear priorities, and with specific targeting of technologies towards the solution of health problems of the majority.

---

* Deputy Director-General, World Health Organization, Geneva, Switzerland.

Thirdly, that an appropriate infrastructure should be developed and maintained. This concept presupposes the national ability to identify, evaluate, adapt and absorb technologies to be transferred.

Fourthly, that adequate manpower should be trained, as scientists, engineers and managerial staff. Twinning and networking arrangements have been widely proposed and explored.

Fifthly, that equipment-related requirements should be carefully assessed and managed. Of particular concern here are not only problems of maintenance, but also the capacity to adapt, modify and produce equipment under economically viable conditions.

Let me turn now to the constraints. We often hear that foremost in the range is lack of political will, whether the will to decide, or the will to think about the future, in addition to the chronic "fire-fighting". Let us assume that such a will can be made to exist. It would have to co-exist with the day-to-day needs of policy management, which would absorb most resources, both time and others.

A further assumption would have to be that sufficient human resources can be spared to set up competently a coherent picture of national needs. This implies two things: an intelligent situation-analysis and an informed comprehension of current and emerging technological possibilities. These two conditions are far from simple and can by no means result from decrees.

It can therefore be argued that under "political will" is subsumed a complex developmental process in which collective and synergistic efforts are essential to promote social, economic and technological welfare.

In the health sector, some of the major constraints naturally relate to costs.

The United States of America, which is at the cutting edge of technological development, spends 12% of its gross national product on health, double the rate of two other industrial countries such as Japan and the United Kingdom, and quadruple that of many poor countries. So, with more than $2000 per capita, can the United States afford the new medical technologies? Well, even here, the cost constraints are evident. It has been estimated that the cost of heart transplants for the 800,000 Americans who could benefit from the procedure would alone represent 10% of GNP. Likewise, if in ten years' time the cost of AIDS treatment were to be the same as it is today, it alone would absorb 10% of GNP. Also, it must be remembered that at present 30% of all health care costs are incurred during the last six months of life.

Clearly, if technology transfer is to have a positive impact on Third World health, a new model of health care delivery and health system development needs to be constructed. In this respect, past experience would appear to be of limited use, and more research is obviously needed.

Perhaps a little elaboration would be in order. It is readily understood that society does not have access to unlimited resources in order to satisfy its needs. A process of selection and exclusion is unavoidable. The market-system model, whereby those who cannot afford goods and services do not get them, is clearly unacceptable for the health sector, since it would contravene the principle of social equity.

At the same time, leaving the complex decision-making process to a politicized techno-bureaucracy would be equally undesirable. For example, what would be the strength of criteria ruling the allocation of resources for early detection of cancer, for injury-related therapy, for emergency care?

The cost for all of these choices is technology-dependent. Given the current cost of technology and the range of perceived societal needs, it cannot be said that the problem of technological "affordability" has been solved in the North.

The South suffers from the worst of both worlds—not only because each country has its own North, but also because the morbidity pattern in the South is quickly adding the diseases of affluence to its burden of under-development ills.

At this point, I hope that the case for methodological research can be accepted without much controversy. The search for new methods of resource allocation, of determining and ranking priorities, is research of a strategic nature. Strategic decisions are those that derive from a global understanding of a given situation; yet they take judicious advantage of specific temporal and spatial features to achieve a high-level objective. Thus, a country wishing to expand its internal-revenue base will decide to give a 10-year tax break to specific new industries in a particular region. Far from being paradoxical, the decision, if properly followed through, may lead to industrial prosperity and subsequent tax revenues from large segments of the population. A similar line of action can be pursued in the field of health.

If interventions x and y are major determinants of health, if there is a latent period of n years before the health effects of x can be perceived, and if the efficacy of y depends on x, then it would be a mistake not to wait n years before intervening with y. How often have costly interventions been abandoned as failures because this cardinal strategic principle has been violated!

The problem, of course, is that many of the "if-then" relationships have not been elucidated—a clear case for pursuing methodological research of a strategic nature.

For example, WHO Member States have accepted primary health care as the way to achieve health for all. Its very success is likely to produce an increased need for secondary and tertiary care, because of improved survival and its consequential burden of morbidity. What methods do we have to advise various countries, various regions, about the redeployment of their technological resources within specific time-frames, say, 10, 20, 50 years?

If the incidence of diarrhoeal diseases and acute respiratory infections drops by 50%, then the infant mortality rate will drop by a related percentage. If so, then the likely occurrence of conditions x, y, z will rise according to spatio-temporal scenarios yet to be determined and evaluated. The necessary technological resources to cope with such conditions, their probable costs over time, and the methodology for obtaining such information on a large scale are all matters that have never been explored.

This brings us to the specific role of WHO in technology and research.

Although in many instances WHO is able to play the role of clearing-house for information, a role recognized and appreciated by many, it is often true that we suffer from important gaps in our knowledge. These gaps relate to our frequent inability to rank priorities on a rational basis, or even to comprehend the hierarchical relationship between various health problems, and that between them and other socioeconomic problems. For example, which is a priority with regard to resource allocation: to treat infectious diseases or to prevent them? The decision is often made easy by the fact that certain technologies are reasonably cheap and permit both approaches (e.g., immunization and oral rehydration). However, it is often true that infrastructural technologies which would prevent a disease or a group of diseases (say, waterborne parasitic infestations) are very expensive. The result is a chronic financial drain on the health services for therapeutic care, which might contain but not solve the particular health problem. Naturally, alternatives have been proposed, designed for changing the behaviour and lifestyle of populations at risk. However, if this is to be successful, it needs to have a firm scientific basis, and it would also require research and technological contributions. Moreover, what may be esoteric technology today could become available to everybody tomorrow.

The intricate nature of all these problems is illustrated by the complex linkages between the environment (both physical and socio-cultural), economics (as regards policies and determinants) and individual human beings. It is what makes the formulation of rational health policies a very difficult task. It is for this reason that policies may frequently appear subjective, arbitrary, or at least ill-conceived. This should provide us with a case for doing more policy-oriented research, to help decision-makers in their difficult task. We should spare no effort to seek new methods to this end—for example, in the field of information technology. In other words, problem assessment is a problem in itself, for which rigorous scientific methodology is required and where the research establishment must play a key role. Needless to say, we in WHO must help and promote the development of such methodologies.

Technology has often been defined as the application of scientific knowledge to practical tasks. If we consider planning as one of the major tasks of health policy-makers, it would be legitimate to enquire what are the technologies available to them? Are they computers? These are no more than instruments. Charting techniques? These are no more than recipes and productivity tools. No, the real technologies should enable a health planner to implement his programmes with a high degree of predictability. They constitute, of course, a whole complex of skills and human knowledge. This is where we need human resource development, where we need imagination and innovation. Here, as elsewhere, research and development is inseparable from technological development.

How can we in WHO help?

The traditional role of the Organization in scientific and technical cooperation is well-known. Tens of thousands of scientists collaborate with WHO in several thousand institutions throughout the world. Many of them take part in the daily life of the Organization, shaping up its collective "state-of-the-art" expertise through meetings, workshops and seminars. Equally well known is the vast network of WHO collaborating centres, which provide research and training facilities, and consultative and bibliographical services, as well as biological references and stand-ard-setting functions.

Beyond this traditional role, it may be opportune to consider new perspectives for international collaboration. It is indisputable that science and technology are moving fast and that, despite the variety of disciplines and programmes represented in WHO, the Organization may not always be in an optimal position to capture the benefits of science for solving problems of world health.

Firstly, there is a need not only of analysis, but also of synthesis.

The greater specialization and verticalization characteristic of contemporary science should not lead us into tubular vision and fragmentation.

There is scope for broadening the spectrum of scientific advice which is provided to WHO. In this respect the Advisory Committee on Health Research has wisely recommended the establishment of a new body, related to it, which would operate flexibly to monitor and forecast new scientific and technological developments.

Secondly, there is a need to strengthen the relationship between WHO and scientific institutions throughout the world. In addition to the existing formal and informal programme-related networks, problem-related issues ought to be addressed, in the sense to which I referred earlier, paying due attention to training and to methodological research. This requires a medium- to long-term approach and high institutional stability. Perhaps the types of institutional arrangements set up by other United Nations bodies could be adapted for WHO purposes.

Two specific situations must be distinguished here: the regionally-based institutions, whose task would be to upgrade research capacity in geographically defined areas in the South; and the internationally established research institutions, whose role would be to perform advanced studies for solving major health problems afflicting the developing countries.

Thirdly, every WHO programme should have the capacity to forecast, or at least anticipate, the types of technological development that are likely to be relevant. The time-horizon should be 10, 20, even 40 years. After all, 40 years have already elapsed since the creation of WHO. This forecasting capacity could only strengthen the technical advice and information which countries expect from the Organization. It could equally strengthen the capacity of countries for setting up groups for technology assessment and technology adaptation.

In concluding, Mr Chairman, dear colleagues, I would stress that technology transfer is not only about goods and productive capacity; it is also about the capacity to think and to innovate. Research and development, research training, and even general education, are essential elements of this capacity in this problem. I hope that so long as we keep in mind all these aspects WHO will be able to make a decisive contribution.

THE ROLE OF FORECASTERS IN HEALTH TECHNOLOGY TRANSFER

Henry Danielsson*

I have been asked to talk about forecasting and its role in technology transfer but also about, and with emphasis on, recent advances in biomedical research and their possible impact on future health care. It seems natural to begin with advances in biomedical research and end with mechanisms of forecasting.

The expansion of knowledge through biomedical research during the last 25–30 years has been remarkable, as has the use of this knowledge in practical health care. Research in many disciplines, ranging from biochemistry to different clinical specialties, has contributed to this knowledge, but the most important and far-reaching contributions have undoubtedly come from molecular biology. From the discovery of the double-stranded DNA (deoxyribonucleic acid) and the genetic code, to recombinant DNA techniques, molecular biology has advanced at a pace and in a way that nobody could have foreseen 30 years ago. The tools of molecular biology are now becoming indispensable in many areas of biomedicine.

Perhaps the most significant breakthroughs so far from research in molecular biology have occurred in genetics. Genetics has become molecular genetics. From a primarily morphological discipline, genetics today describes its findings in terms of molecular biology. The number of structurally defined genes increases rapidly. With present and projected efforts in mapping and sequencing the human genome, it is not unreasonable to assume that most of the 100,000 genes in the human genome will be known by the year 2000. Just as important as knowing the structure of the genes will be knowledge about the rest of the DNA. It can be calculated that the genes account for something like 10 % of the 3 billion nucleotides in the DNA. What does the rest of the DNA do? Today, little is known about this.

The impact of advances in molecular genetics on our understanding of many diseases is becoming increasingly evident. An important role of genetics has already been established in many common diseases. Increasing knowledge about the human genome will provide very much improved tools for diagnosis and prevention, sometimes even treatment, of disease. As an example of a genetic component in a common disease I would mention Alzheimer disease. Evidence has been presented to indicate the involvement of defects in chromosome 21 in cases of Alzheimer disease. However, it is likely that Alzheimer disease, like many others, is triggered by a combination of several factors, viz. a predisposing genetic defect, environment and the ageing process itself.

---

* Professor, Swedish Medical Research Council, Stockholm, Sweden.

Similar findings have been made with respect to some cancers. In this case, oncogenes play an important role. Oncogenes were discovered some years ago in studies of virus-induced cancers. Today, some 50 different oncogenes are known. Oncogenes code for a variety of proteins such as protein kinases, growth factors and growth-factor receptors. They are present in normal cells and are involved in regulation of normal growth. When they are deregulated or are altered by mutations, they may cause malignant transformations. An example is bladder cancer in man, which is associated with a point mutation in the cellular *ras* gene, resulting in a single amino-acid exchange. Recent work indicates that the activation of a single oncogene does not by itself result in transformation and tumour development—the cooperation of other genes is necessary. A working hypothesis is that other genes may control the expression of oncogenes. In this context, the anti-oncogenes should be mentioned. An example of an anti-oncogene is the retinoblastoma gene (Rb 1). The product of this gene prevents tumour formation.

Even if advances in molecular biology in recent years have been rapid and have sometimes unexpected repercussions it should be borne in mind that much other biomedical research has made important contributions that will lead to improved health care in the coming years. The advance of immunology has been particularly noteworthy. The most spectacular single advance in recent years is the hybridoma technique for obtaining monoclonal antibodies. The increasing knowledge of the mechanisms by which our immune system functions will provide additional tools for our fight against infectious diseases of various kinds and against cancer. Recent studies of the regulation of the immune system justify these expectations. The intense research into the interleukins, polypeptides that regulate the immune system, has led to the isolation of eight different peptides. Some of these have been prepared by recombinant DNA technology and have entered clinical trials for treatment of certain cancers, primarily leukemia.

Neurobiology and neurochemistry are other areas that have progressed beyond expectations. The analysis of the mechanisms of nerve-impulse transmission in both the central and the peripheral nervous system has provided results that have found applications in treatment of disease and will continue to do so. In recent years a number of neuropeptides—up to now about 40—have been detected and structurally determined. It has been suggested that disturbances in neuropeptide formation may cause dysfunction of the nervous system.

The developments in clinical sciences have been substantial, with respect to both diagnostic and therapeutic procedures. To a large extent, these advances have depended, and will depend, on advances in basic research, not least in molecular biology and immunology. It should be emphasized that in some instances the advances have built on techniques in sciences outside those normally included in biomedical sciences, such as physical and mathematical sciences. Generally, the advances in diagnostic procedures have been more rapid than those in therapeutic procedures. However, the latter should not be underestimated. Suffice it to mention that in the developed countries 50% of many common cancers are cured today, that the advent of artificial joints has changed in a remarkable way the lives of those afflicted by various forms of arthritis, and that the transplantation of organs, not least kidneys, has resulted in drastic changes for those normally condemned to premature death.

The following are examples of probable or possible improvements in diagnosis, treatment and prevention of some common diseases thanks to developments in biomedical research.

Infectious diseases

Infectious diseases, whether of bacterial, parasitic or viral origin, can be considered in a worldwide perspective to be the most important group of diseases to combat. At the present state of knowledge this combat is likely to be more successful in a 10 to 15 year perspective than that directed at many other diseases. The major factors behind this supposition are the advances in molecular biology and immunology. Knowledge about the chemistry of micro-organisms and the mechanisms of their replication offers possibilities to produce vaccines specific for important structures responsible for infectivity of the micro-organisms. At the same time, this way of attacking the problems of vaccine production decreases or eliminates unwanted side-effects of vaccines. Recombinant DNA technology has provided an instrument to prepare immunogenic material at reasonable cost. A particular advantage of this technology is that deletion mutants lacking certain virulent genes can be prepared. These mutants will be antigenic but will be safer than vaccines prepared according to procedures currently used. Another possibility for vaccine production involves utilization of subunits or components of micro-organisms. Such vaccines will contain parts that are antigenic but lack components that may cause infections or other unwanted side-effects.

With regard to parasitic diseases, and the example of malaria, it can be assumed that vaccines will contain proteins from different stages of the evolution of the malaria parasite. By such a design it will be possible to attack the parasite at different stages of its life-cycle. However, it is an enormous task to delineate which structures constitute the major antigens. Research dealing with malaria has progressed the farthest and there are well-founded hopes that an effective malaria vaccine will be available within the next five to seven years.

Cardiovascular diseases

Cardiovascular diseases are the foremost cause of death and disability in the developed countries and constitute an increasing problem in developing countries. While the prospects of making great progress in the elimination of many infectious diseases in the coming 10–15 years are good, those of a decrease in morbidity and mortality in cardiovascular diseases in the near future must be considered less favourable. Unquestionably, risk factors such as high fat-intake and smoking have been defined and suitable changes of life-style are likely to have an impact. It seems that the very considerable efforts that have gone into research into cardiovascular diseases is starting to pay off. There is convincing evidence that decreasing cholesterol levels in serum leads to reduced risk of coronary infarction. Very large multicentre studies have shown this in a convincing way. Further, the basic research on regulation of cholesterol synthesis in the liver is providing new insights into possible mechanisms to influence cholesterol metabolism.

A new approach to the causation of cardiovascular diseases, different from that related to diet and life-style factors, involves the thrombocytes. Recent research has shown that aggregation of thrombocytes—an early phase of blood coagulation and thrombus formation—is regulated by the interplay between the arachnidonic acid metabolites, prostacyclin and thromboxanes—the former preventing aggregation, the latter stimulating aggregation. It is conceivable that a change of the normal process of thrombocyte aggregation may be important in cardiovascular disease. If so, one can visualize a treatment modality based on inhibitors or stimulators of prostacyclin and thromboxanes. Aspirin, i.e. acetylsalicylic acid, has been shown to inhibit the biosynthesis of prostacyclin and thromboxanes. Several large clinical trials have been performed in which the possible benefit of low-dose aspirin in preventing coronary infarction and stroke has been examined. The results indicate that such treatment is of value.

Yet, a long-range aim should be prevention, and present knowledge is insufficient for successful prevention. However, prevention can not be the sole solution. Evidence is accumulating that there is also a genetic predisposition to cardiovascular disease.

Cancers

In developed countries cancer is responsible for some 25% of all deaths and is thus the second most common cause of death. In developing countries, where life expectancy is shorter, cancer causes 5–10% of all deaths. It has been calculated that cancer incidence at present increases by about 5% per year. About 65% of all cancers occur in the age groups above 65 years of age, and the average age of the population is increasing gradually. Survival patterns and prognosis for several common cancers have improved over the years and five-year survival for many common cancers is now at least 50%. The best results by far have been achieved in cancers of childhood. Several cancers of older children and young adults are also being treated with good results.

In recent years methods of early detection have been developed and clear effects in decreased morbidity and mortality have been demonstrated. Prevention plays a significant role. Elimination of tobacco smoking would be a very important step in decreasing incidence of cancer. Correlations between composition of diet and incidence of cancer have been demonstrated, e.g. in colon cancer, but much more needs to be known about relationships between diet and cancer.

Psychiatric and neurological diseases

Progress in neurobiology promises great hope for better means of treating psychiatric and neurological diseases. The meticulous and painstaking work on clarifying neurotransmission has already provided important tools for treatment of disease. A classical example by now is Parkinson's disease, which is characterized by deficient production of dopamine. Administration of dopa—a precursor of dopamine—for this disease is a standard procedure today.

Many psychiatric diseases are associated with disturbances in neurotransmitter production or metabolism. Recent examples are depressive diseases, which can be associated with decreased serotonin production, and Alzheimer disease, which is associated with deficient acetylcholine production.

Basic research findings with implications for therapy are those concerned with growth and repair of the nervous system. In recent years a number of growth factors have been identified. Also, such factors as gangliosides have been shown to play a role in nerve growth and repair. The application of this knowledge to treatment of neurodegenerative diseases and injury is foreseen within the coming 10 years.

Knowledge of the biochemical changes in psychiatric and neurological diseases provides tools for substitution therapy and drug design, Indeed, it is to be assumed that, as knowledge about the mechanisms of function of the nervous system increases, instruments are provided for the design of increasingly efficient drugs.

Technology assessment and technology transfer

The results of biomedical and other research are continuously applied to both the established and the emerging health-care technologies. There is an increasingly recognized need to assess the safety and efficacy of these technologies. This field of research and development, the assessment of health-care technologies, is growing rapidly. Part of these activities should deal with future health-care technologies.

One of the few studies that have been carried out on future health-care technologies is that commissioned by the Steering Committee on Future Health Scenarios, a Royal Commission advising the Government of the Netherlands on long-term developments in health and health care. The study was carried out between 1986 and 1988 and involved a survey of the opinions of hundreds of experts concerning possible and probable developments in their area of expertise and the impact of these developments on health care. In a second phase a number of specific areas were selected for in-depth study: neurosciences, especially the regeneration of nervous tissue; lasers, especially their application in treatment of coronary artery disease; biotechnology, especially the development of new vaccines; genetic screening; computer-assisted medical imaging, especially the case of picture archiving and communications systems; and home-care technologies. The study on lasers in the treatment of coronary artery disease was extended to the preparation of a rather complete scenario, including economic assessments.

A major conclusion of the project was that an early-warning system was needed, i.e. a system that would monitor research developments and their possible influence on health care and health care systems.

The desirability of including in national systems of assessment of health-care technology a continuous monitoring of advances in research related to health care has been discussed in several countries. With regard to both assessment of health-care technology and monitoring of research advances, there is a need for international collaboration, which would be facilitated by the creation of national focal points. It seems natural that WHO should initiate a similar activity to support an efficient transfer of technologies to the developing countries.

THE PERSPECTIVE OF TECHNOLOGY BROKERS IN HEALTH TECHNOLOGY TRANSFER

David Dichter*

No one would deny that there has been a thorough change of attitudes in the past several years as to what sort of role profit-making companies ought to have in the development process. After nearly three decades in which governments and international aid agencies have looked primarily toward the public sector for ways of promoting economic and social development in Third-World countries, many of these countries are now willing to accept much greater participation by private business firms, and also to accord them their due share of importance where national development priorities are concerned.

Within the context of private business assisting in the development process, the transfer of technology is widely regarded as being a key element for unleashing economic growth, principally by increasing productivity, helping to raise income levels, and creating new employment opportunities. Recently, attention has been focused on the role that individual companies can play (particularly small and medium-sized firms) in transferring a wide range of production technologies and requisite managerial know-how and marketing experience to their counterparts in various Third-World countries.

Enterprise-to-enterprise transfer as opposed to government-to-government assistance programmes is increasingly being seen as perhaps a more realistic and effective way to accelerate the industrial development of the Third World. By having one firm supply another with relevant technical assistance and managerial skills and advising it on what type of production equipment to acquire, technology transfer can be accomplished in a more efficient and effective way than by funnelling scarce foreign aid resources solely through government channels.

The traditional approach to technical training and industrial development programmes has been to identify a need for certain skills in a developing country (or simply suppose there must be a need), send an expert to the country to give a course, have the government concerned select people to take the course, and conduct the training programme, at the end of which everyone separated. The foreign development expert returned home or moved to other similar projects in the region, and the government-selected trainees were scattered about. Many of them never used the skills learned; some complained that the skills were not applicable in their own countries. Others could not find work with the skills taught to them.

This type of approach has been classic. Its limitations and inefficiencies are obvious. Because such programmes bypassed, virtually from beginning to end, the business sector (perhaps the best determiner of what

---

* Director, Technology for the People, Geneva, Switzerland.

skills are needed in the market) and were often conducted on a government-to-government basis, totally unrelated to marketplace conditions, there was inevitably a certain "unreality" in the entire exercise. Apparently also, there was little or no incentive to follow through on such programmes, and as a result all of the parties went their separate ways at the conclusion of such projects.

Early in the post-colonial period, the most significant technology transfers were made to developing countries by subsidiaries of transnational corporations. Technology was often purchased or licensed separately, either as equipment or in the form of trademarks and designs. There was considerable copying of production equipment as well.

Business had not yet come to be recognised by host governments as a vehicle for improving human welfare—much less as a crucial factor in the overall development process. As a consequence, bilateral foreign-aid agencies and multilateral development banks did little or nothing to assist technology transfer, largely overlooking that geared specifically to small and medium-sized enterprises.

At the same time, developing countries were becoming increasingly aware of the valuable applications of new technology—not only for industrial growth, but also for alleviating unemployment, boosting trade and repaying foreign debts. They began to realise that technology might be at least as important as capital accumulation and creation of physical infrastructure.

However, because many of them wanted to be free to pursue their own goals of greater technological independence and self-sufficiency, all sorts of objections began to be raised about foreign firms seeking equity investments or licensing arrangements for their industrial property. During this early post-colonial period a mutually incriminating and often acrimonious dialogue followed, eventually leading many Third-World countries to enact complex licensing controls, rigorous royalty arrangements and tough restrictions on joint ventures. Foreign firms—including small and medium-sized ones—were required to invest substantial amounts of capital as a guarantee of "good faith" and to ensure the firm's long-term cooperation and participation in the host country's industrial growth.

While policies such as these are understandable, given past circumstances, particularly where the fear of the large multinational corporations was concerned, they are now coming under increasing criticism as being shortsighted and inappropriate. Measures are being taken in a number of developing countries to facilitate the transfer to local firms of a wide range of production technologies that they deem important to their development. Investment laws are being modified, especially in the amount of "up-front" capital required, to encourage many more foreign small or medium-sized companies to share their technology and managerial know-how with prospective collaborators.

It was at the beginning of this more relaxed "pro-business" environment—some 12 years ago—that Technology for the People (TFTP) was launched. Established under Geneva Cantonal law as a non-profit, international service organization (it has since obtained tax-free status), it saw as its goal to use or obtain contracts from donor governments and agencies to directly support technology transfer and international trade on a company-to-company basis. Having worked for a number of years in developing countries in government-to-government technical assistance programmes, the founder of the organization came to realize that these programmes did not normally provide the proper incentives to get the job done. What was needed in his estimation was an element of profit to become the driving force, with small and medium-sized business firms as the vital partners in the development process.

From the outset, TFTP has taken the position that: 1) business and development interests are compatible; 2) commercially-oriented technology transfer arrangements between enterprises are a very effective way to help improve living standards in developing countries; 3) profit has a vital role in stimulating motivation and also helps to ensure better project management and accountability; and 4) the entrepreneur is the key element in the development process; whether in an industrialized or a developing country, it is the entrepreneur's integrity, imagination, and dynamism that will ensure the success of the business deal.

The organization's first practical efforts in trying to increase direct contacts between Third-World businessmen and commercial firms from the industrialized nations was to sponsor a series of international technology transfer fairs in different parts of the world. They were conceived as a sort of "one-stop shopping place", especially for Third-World business people seeking to acquire specific production technologies, and also as a convenient place to conduct on-the-spot negotiations. At each of the four fairs held to date: Geneva, Mexico City, Manila and Budapest, the focus was on what small and medium-sized companies could offer one another.

As a result of its trade-fair experience, TFTP began to focus its efforts more and more on direct intermediary work for company-to-company technology transfer. During the past seven years it has worked to transfer technology from European firms, primarily Swiss, to individual companies throughout South and South-East Asia. More recently it has been laying the groundwork for a comprehensive "south-to-south" transfer of production technologies from small and medium-sized Asian firms to prospective collaborators in a number of sub-Saharan African countries.

Interestingly enough, one of the principal problems the organization has had in extending its technology brokering activities is that profit was, and continues to be, a difficult concept for many United Nations officials, as well as for bureaucrats of both donor and developing countries, to accept. Apparently, many of these officials are still unwilling to support the thesis that by making a profit the Third-World businessman is actually increasing income in his country, creating new jobs and in the process generating surplus capital for the additional purchase of foreign technology.

TFTP has also taken a very decisive stand on the issue of appropriate technology, and what it sees as a considerable waste of resources on the part of universities and development-oriented research institutes in Western Europe and the United States in trying to create the perfect mud stove or pump for developing countries. It is the organization's view that, when this "new technology" is tried in the field, it is often rejected by the local people, even if it is given away. The reason is, in TFTP's estimation, that the appropriate technology people chose to bypass regular commercial channels. They did not take into account market demands or the requirements for setting up an effective commercial distribution network. Instead, they focused their attention almost exclusively on the supply side, rather ignoring market realities and refusing to collaborate with local merchants.

If anything, the experience which TFTP staff have acquired in the past decade has reinforced their position about the importance of intermediation in the transfer of technology. However, they are under no illusions that their role as technology brokers has been anything unique or new. Indeed, banks, patent experts, law firms, and consulting organizations have all been playing active roles for many years in facilitating such arrangements. Especially in the more advanced industrial countries, this has included obtaining capital, equipment and special technology resources in putting together a particular business deal.

What is relatively new in the technology brokering field is the work being carried on by TFTP and several other specialized consulting organizations to serve the interests of primarily small and medium-sized companies willing to offer their technology and know-how to Third World firms. This involves not only companies in the industrialized countries offering their know-how and production technology to prospective Third-World collaborators, but also, in the more technically advanced developing nations, firms willing to transfer their technology on a "south-to-south" basis.

Experience has shown that most small and medium-sized enterprises often lack international experience and expertise, and must incur relatively high front-end costs to gain access to international markets or sources of supply. Under the circumstances, they usually require the services of an outside intermediary (organization or person) who can act as both a catalyst and a facilitator to help bring the parties together, structure the venture, and assist in bringing it to fruition.

Although there is certainly no set game-plan in brokering such business ventures—since usually every deal worked on is totally different from any other—a few areas can be listed where the expertise of such persons is likely to be offered to client firms. These include:

(a) Locating technology suppliers and in certain cases the required equity sources
(b) Arranging technical research and marketing studies
(c) Coordinating the activities of the participating firms
(d) Organizing any product testing or field trials which might be required
(e) Helping draw up the most appropriate legal instruments, and then joining the negotiations as the "objective third party" to help finalize the deal.

However, when it comes to arranging a transfer of technology in which initially commercial considerations are not in the forefront, but which, nevertheless, is deemed very important by host governments, UN agencies and development aid organisations, because of "development considerations", then the broker's role takes on special significance. In such instances brokers may even be responsible for initiating projects, since often they not only are well-informed about the technical needs of many developing countries (and the best local firms with which to work), but also know where to find the most suitable and cost-effective companies that can provide such technology.

Speaking for myself, I find this aspect of technology brokering to be one of the most challenging and professionally satisfying activities in which I have ever been engaged. Not only is it exciting because of the wide range of production technologies which one can offer firms in developing nations from prospective colleagues in other countries, but if one is successful in one's efforts, then the results obtained—in increased productivity and job creation—are likely to be quite substantial.

I have been privileged these past nine months to work with certain WHO technical staff in trying to find a cost-effective way of producing a basic X-ray system which not only meets WHO's stringent technical and performance requirements, but at the same time can be used widely in many of the world's least developed countries.

Since price was obviously a key factor in helping to popularize such a system, a decision was taken early on to try to identify a competent firm in one of the newly industrialized countries in South and South-East Asia. Such a company had to be capable of handling many of the project's technical requirements, and also its production costs and profit expectations had to be in line with with the projected free-on-board price of such a unit.

Work is going forward on this important project in cooperation with an outstanding X-ray equipment manufacturing company in a developing country, and this company in turn is collaborating with a leading radiological equipment firm in an industrialized country.

However, most Third-World business-men are unaware of the utility of the services of intermediaries. Many of their firms are unable to evaluate the costs and benefits of new business opportunities, and are therefore reluctant to pay fees for professional assistance during the early planning and evaluation stages of a project. Also, they have difficulty in assigning an explicit value to the role and the remuneration of the technology broker. In contrast, they are accustomed to paying for legal and accounting, and even engineering, services, which relate to the more traditional needs of the enterprise. It is not surprising therefore to find that such intermediation (especially in the least developed countries) is sporadic and normally offered only as a secondary service by service organizations.

Other types of intermediaries such as investment bankers, marketing organizations, trading companies and some technology suppliers often choose to relate their compensation to the percentage of sales or income generated by the project.

Since the concept of paying for such services is alien to most Third-World countries, somebody must be found who will pay for special technology brokering work and its related expenses. Donors can, and should, look to such specializied intermediaries as a vehicle for helping to achieve important development objectives, especially for the acquisition, adoption and utilization of new production technology. It is unreasonable to expect such intermediaries to fund the expenses, perform the work, bear the risk, and wait perhaps for years for a return that may never come. However, it is only very recently that the development-aid community has seen the need to engage the services of such technology brokers as catalysts in the development process.

It is understandable, therefore, why so many potentially important development-oriented technology-transfer projects have never been realized. Other constraints involve foreign government restrictions, such as local content regulations, the need for direct foreign investment as a precondition for collaboration, and the difficulties involved in repatriating earnings. Thus, it is not surprising that many small and medium-sized enterprises in both industrialized and the more advanced Third-World countries display a "stay at home" attitude and are reluctant to venture into a realm that is truly foreign and fraught with unknowns.

The skills which an effective technology broker must bring to bear in the successful pursuit of his profession may be summarized as follows:

(1) Successful client-development: This involves the identification and cultivation of a number of potential clients with active or passive interest in supplying or receiving production technology. It is the process whereby technology brokers properly organize and "sell" such ventures so that enterprises can overcome their natural resistance to new ventures. Unless the intermediary can convince the participating firms of the likely results and that the risk is manageable, the firms will take no further action.

(2) The ability to generate credibility and trust among prospective clients: Technology brokers must be able to demonstrate that they are acting in the best interests of each of the participating firms and apply sound business ethics throughout the entire life of the project.

(3) Data analysis and using technology networks: A good technology broker invests a lot of time in building up his company contacts and information sources, and also seeks ways and means of creating business linkages between potential suppliers and users of suitable production technologies.

(5) Access to financial resources: Although technology brokers may not have direct access to financial resources, at least they can realistically advise clients about potential funding sources, including development finance institutions, banks, and government aid organisations.

Thus, a good intermediary is a person who not only is well-versed in the intricacies of joint-venturing, licensing, subcontracting and other forms of international transactions, but also can provide the necessary "hands-on" and personalized assistance to the different participants to successfully broker a transfer of technology. Above all, the good intermediary must have the patience and fortitude to stick with it even when, for months at a time, seemingly no progress is being made.

THE CONSULTANT'S ROLE IN IN TECHNOLOGY TRANSFER

John F. Moore*

I. Introduction

In technology transfer the consultant can play two rôles: direct and indirect. The direct rôle provides, through the consultant's own staff, capabilities which either party to the transfer may lack. These may include management, design, training, and documentation. In the indirect rôle, the generalist consultant acts as a broker, obtaining knowledge or negotiating participation from third parties, such as other specialist consultants. However, the most valuable contribution of an experienced consultant is less obvious: it is to assure both parties that all significant factors have been considered in advance, in order to minimize the likelihood of unpleasant surprises.

While technology transfer has sometimes been defined to include the importation and use of a new material, drug, or product, this paper is directed toward those cases where the user country intends to produce the new technology. This paper provides a list and description of some of those factors important in technology transfer between nations and regions. The list may also become a framework within which individual transfers of technology can better be accomplished.

In the first section, some of the key factors are defined. In subsequent sections, different cases are considered in more detail, with comments on where the consultant can help.

Instead of emphasizing the consultant, the emphasis is placed on the transfer process.

A. Definitions: The Ingredients

1. Skills
This topic refers to the human abilities that are required, ranging from the simplest levels of assembly to the highest levels of design and management. However, it should be recognized that technology transfer cannot ignore certain other skills that are *not* directly involved in the transfer itself. For example, governmental and educational skill levels will be extremely important for the long-term success of any project.

2. Materials
The term "materials" encompasses the entire range from raw materials through processed materials, including manufactured parts and components.

---

* Director, Bio-Imaging Research, Inc. Lincolnshire, Illinois, USA.

144

3. Methods

While this topic has some overlap with Skills, it refers primarily to the availability of machinery and equipment to support various aspects of the manufacturing process.

4. Participants

In this paper, the provider of technology is referred to as the "provider", and the country or region benefiting from the transfer is called the "user".

5. Finance

We recognize that the availability of financing is a *sine qua non* for any technology transfer. Funding may come from the provider, the user, private organizations, companies or international organizations. The form of these funds is not critical to the success of the transfer as long as the amounts are adequate, and as long as the participants' *quid pro quo* (such as royalties, interest, or other obligations) to the funding source do not represent a burden to the economy of the user or to the project itself. We add the caution that many projects end up requiring 50% to 100% funding more than estimated initially. For that reason, a funding source with adequate reserves is to be preferred. However, since details of funding deserve a full-scale treatment separate from the technology, they will not be discussed further in this paper.

B. Definitions: The Environments

Classification of countries or regions into categories is somewhat arbitrary. In one sense, there is almost a continuous spectrum, from those with the least skills, materials and methods to those with the most. This spectrum may actually be nonlinear, in the sense that one country may be more advanced in some areas while another country is more advanced in others. There also may be wide variations within a single country. Nevertheless, in order to deal with specifics, we have defined three main environments for technology transfer, while recognizing that there will always be borderline cases between them.

1. The Technology Reservoir Areas

This refers to those countries which have been investing time and money in new technologies for the longest period. These "reservoir" areas have often amassed enough skills, materials, methods and finances so that they not only are sufficient to drive their own further progress, but also represent resources that can be of substantial benefit to the other parts of the entire world. Examples include many nations of Western Europe, North America, and the north-western Pacific rim.

2. The Active Transceiver Areas

These nations represent those with the greatest degrees of technological ferment. They are simultaneously engaged in three levels of activity:

enhancing their technology and product base through their own efforts, acquiring additional technology from reservoir nations, and adding to their trade by providing technology and service to the remaining nations. This intermediate position—being both a receiver and a transmitter, coupled with their intense activity, gives them a key role in technology transfer. Borrowing a term from the field of communications, we will call these "transceiver" areas. Examples might include India, Israel, and several countries in South America and the south-west Pacific rim.

3. The Greatest Potential
These remaining nations and areas are those which will function primarily as users of technology transfer. They are often characterized by high ratios of population to food and financing. However, they represent the areas where technology transfer has the greatest potential for improving the standard of living. The are therefore referred to as "potential" areas.

II. Case A: Reservoir to transceiver

In this first case, we consider technology transfer from the reservoir nations (those with the greatest skills, materials and methods) to those in an intermediate status, the transceivers. One of the key characteristics of this class of transfer is that it will usually deal with higher technology products than in transfer to potential nations, whether from reservoir or transceiver. For this reason, it is often of greater interest to members of the financial community, who see obvious opportunities for profit and growth without excessive risk. It is therefore less likely to require assistance from international agencies. It also requires less participation from consultants, as both parties are likely to possess most of the management skills and a good general level of technical and industrial skills. The consultant's direct rôle may be limited to providing specialist expertise; it also may help indirectly by guiding the parties in coordinating their relations with the many (and often conflicting) government agencies that are common in reservoir and transceiver countries.

Note, however, that these transfers do relatively less to improve the world's living conditions than those which will be considered later.

A. Skills

In general, the transceivers will possess enough of the skills in the categories listed below to enable them to readily understand the knowledge that is to be transferred from the reservoir. Furthermore, their educational systems may already be producing a larger ratio of technically trained individuals to their overall economy than is the case in the reservoir nations. This often means that there is substantial technological underemployment in the transceiver nations. This offers an advantage: the length of time required to transfer technology will be shorter, as these well-trained but underemployed individuals need only the practical hands-on experience rather than the entire education process.

1. Management
In most transceiver countries, the principles and skills of organization management are already known. The main management-related items that may be transferred from the reservoir country have to do with increased use of computers as management tools, and (in some cases) the reorientation of the management structure in the user country to fit the special needs of a particular project. However, management personnel in the provider country must recognize that certain principles, practices, and habits in the user country may represent a long tradition that differs from their own. In that case, the consultant can recommend and perform joint study of the organizational differences in order to assess whether those could affect the success of the projects. For example, the user country may have a greater or a smaller dependence on internal communications than the provider country. There may be a different degree of reliance on informal reporting, on group decision-making, etc. The consultant must also analyze whether the management in the user country has comparable responsibilities, and make sure that all the necessary functions are staffed.

Computers should not be put in blindly. Again, the practices of the user must be taken into account, and every effort made to computerize only those operations or data flows that are necessary for the project's success. Well-planned selective computerization is already an important consultant activity, even when technology transfer is not involved.

2. Design
When the user is a transceiver country, it is likely to have all of the necessary theoretical design skills, and will lack only the experience in putting them into practice. There is some danger that provider-country personnel will make the mistake of confusing the lack of practical experience with ignorance. If this is handled badly, it not only will be damaging to the pride of the competent people in the user country, but also can become a source of serious friction. One useful technique is for the scientists, engineers and designers from the provider country to set up design review meetings with their user counterparts. At these meetings, narrative descriptions of the problems which originally occurred in the design being transferred are analyzed with all participants on an equal basis. This process will give examples of what should be avoided by the users, without seeming to denigrate their skills. In those meetings, a consultant can warn of more general problem areas.

3. Documentation
It is unfortunate that higher levels of technology demand higher levels of documentation, with not only increased numbers of drawings but also supplementary documents covering procedures at every level. As in the case of management, we recommend that this documentation burden be introduced gradually. Since the product being transferred will probably

147

be subject to less frequent redesign in the user country than in the provider country, consideration should be given to a simpler level of documentation, particularly with reference to the "change orders" that tend to occur all too frequently. Several consulting firms specialize in rewriting operator and service manuals, including translation, text simplification, and additional graphic or pictorial illustrations.

4. Manufacturing

Since it is difficult for the representatives of the provider country to change the infrastructure of the user's manufacturing environment, it is important to survey the available manufacturing skills and techniques. For example, many transceiver countries have a higher level of skill than reservoir countries in manufacturing areas that do not depend upon extremely large capital equipment items, such as multi-ton presses, chemical milling, high-temperature processes, etc. Product costs can often be reduced by taking advantage of this.

An experienced consultant should be able to tap business and government references, in order to assemble a thorough survey.

4. Distribution/Service

Outside of the city where the transferred product will be manufactured, its successful deployment will be affected by the distribution network. This is especially true of materials, consumables, disposables, and large-volume, low-cost items. Associated factors are distributor business practices, physical security, storage availability and transportation. However, so long as these items are present, deployment can occur—though it may be slower than in the provider country.

The availability of maintenance and repair services—including initial installation for large or complex products—is more important. Without it, all of the other efforts and costs of technology transfer will be wasted.

There are two main types of service: field and depot. Good field service requires an adequate number of mobile trained personnel with suitable test equipment and tools, and a steady flow of spare parts. For some products, depot service is more suitable. It may be less expensive because a central depot will require fewer spare parts, test equipment and tools, and because no personnel travel is required. However, depot service requires that the product be designed so that the user can easily remove defective elements, and snap or plug in the replacement parts sent in exchange. This procedure is better than field service in the undesirable situation where key components or repair processes are available only in the provider country.

In any case, the consultant should carefully study the above factors in the user country to assure the suitability of each technology transfer, and the way in which it will be implemented.

6. End Users

The final necessary step is acceptance of the new technology or product by the end-user, who may be an average consumer, a businessman or a professional. It should not require the end-users to change abruptly their way of life or daily active pattern; nor should it violate community or religious standards. Finally, the general knowledge and educational level of the end-user should be adequate not only to operate the product, but also to understand its significance.

B. Materials

The consultant is ideally suited to analyze the availability of materials in the user country, by compiling data from a range of sources, from trade associations and technical journals to telephone directories and government compilations.

1. Metals
Transceiver country users will generally have a full range of conventional metal alloys, comparable to that of the reservoir-country providers. Exceptions might include alloys with "tailored" grain structure, such as single-crystal casting, or those with exotic ingredients that sell in low quantities even in the provider country. Products or technologies which include such exceptions should be reviewed for possible redesign—a task which may involve a consultant.

2. Chemicals
Chemicals must be looked at from two different viewpoints. First, if it is intended to transfer chemistry-based technology, there may be a problem with regard to piping, reactors and other vessels. What is required in the user country is not only the ability to fabricate these components, but also the ability to test them. For this reason, the decision may be made to fabricate the vessels, etc., in the provider country, and to ship and reassemble them at the receiving site. Alternatively, the provider country may take responsibility for detailed supervision of fabrication in the user country. In that case, it should also take full responsibility for testing. Independent consultants who are specialists in testing are likely to save money in this area.

The other aspect of chemicals is the extent to which they may be required as ingredients for a non-chemical process or product that is being transferred. While many transceiver countries do not have the full breadth of chemical processes that some of the reservoir countries do, they frequently possess the highest level of technology in a few specialized areas, usually based on their own raw-material resources. In such a case, it is desirable to select technology transfer products that can utilize what is already there, in order to avoid forcing the user into dependence on imported materials.

3. Plastics and Composites
Many of the same general comments appply as under Chemicals. Technology transfer that depends on having a capability in ordinary injection molding, sheet plastic forming, or epoxy-fiberglass lay-ups is

likely to be successful, as these techniques will exist or be easily acquired by the user. In the case of more exotic techniques such as carbon-fiber and metal-fiber composites, multi-component extrusions, co-molded items, or the forming of extremely large sections, the facilities within the user country should be reviewed before making a commitment to a technology transfer requiring these techniques.

4. Components

This area represents the greatest potential difficulty, in that the user country should not be forced into relying on importation of high-tech mechanical or electric components such as super-precision ball-bearings or LSI (large-scale integration) microchips. The solution is to return to the design stage of the product being transferred: the design should be modified to take advantage of the level of components that are readily and widely available within the user country. Since the original design team may be committed to their existing design approach, it is frequently faster and less expensive to give the redesign task to a consultant.

For example, one should exercise caution before using the most advanced types of computer or logic chips. Even if their availability is assured, small details in their specifications change frequently, thus jeopardizing the success of the program. This is because it may be too much to expect the user country simultaneously to handle the technology transfer and to change the product design to allow for such changes in component specifications. The same principle applies to mechanical components. Mechanical portions of a product being transferred should be designed to looser tolerances than might be preferred in a reservoir country.

One possible exception is to include computer chips with diagnostic programs stored in read-only memories (ROMs). If these are not part of the normal operation of the product, they can permit service and repair to be performed by less skilled personnel, without reducing operational reliability.

C. Methods

As in the case of materials, consultants can be valuable in assessing the available methods.

1. Fabrication

The product to be transferred should be modified or redesigned to utilize the available techniques, which are likely to be slightly less computer-intensive or capital-equipment-intensive than in the reservoir countries. In some of the transceiver countries, this does not necessarily mean more labor-intensive methods, but simply may direct the use of assembly-line techniques that use a larger number of smaller stations, multiple-mold or multiple-draw fabrication rather than larger single-stage processes, a lower level of automation in machinery, etc. This is not because user personnel cannot handle more complex equipment, but because the

150

equipment represents a liability if its repair requires parts or personnel from the provider country.

2. *Assembly*

The transceiver countries are capable of utilizing automated assembly techniques, but consultants often recommend against using those which are custom designed for a particular product, as servicing may become a limitation. Instead, they recommend general-purpose assembly machinery. Whether or not computer-based systems should be used depends on whether software programming and troubleshooting capability is available near the location where assembly is taking place.

3. *Testing*

Quality assurance on the product being transferred is extremely important, both from the viewpoint of eventual user safety and for the new manufacturer's or country's reputation as a reliable source. For this reason, processes or products should be avoided if they require testing techniques that involve expensive capital equipment, or equipment which cannot readily be serviced and repaired in the user country.

III. Case B: Transceiver to potential

This case, sometimes called "south-to-south transfer", has historically been favored less than transfers from reservoir countries. However, it has several significant advantages which stem from the fact that many transceiver countries have recently progressed from being potential countries, and thus better understand the latter's conditions, standards and problems.

The most important advantage is a higher probability of success. In the last 40 years, there have been all too many examples of reservoir-to-potential transfers that have failed, as discussed below under Case C. Reservoir-country management often expects too much, too soon. Transceiver countries know the need for patience.

Another advantage of the transceiver country as provider is lower cost, through lower salaries, expenses, overhead burden, supplies, etc. Finally, there is the less tangible advantage that, when a potential country acquires appropriate technology, it can do more to alleviate starvation, poverty, disease and debt than any other form of transfer.

In transfers to potential countries, consultants can play a larger part than in the reservoir-to-transceiver case. Not only do they offer relatively more skills, but also there is more opportunity to put together a team. The primary consultant can contact specialist consulting firms (such as personnel, testing, software, etc.), and act as negotiator between all of the organizations that are involved. Consultants from a reservoir country can apply the highest level of skills, computerization, mathematics and management techniques toward planning technology transfer and analyzing its requirements, its individual steps, and its expected results. In this way, they can increase the chances of success, but they must be careful that the plan does not require field use of those high-level techniques in actually executing the transfer.

All of the considerations under Section II (Case A) are relevant to this case as well. To avoid repetition, the following compilation of skills, materials and methods will concentrate on the way in which Case B differs from Case A, and should be taken in conjunction with parallel items discussed previously.

A. Skills

1. Management
Relatively fewer people in potential countries possess the management education and skills required to implement large high-technology start-ups. The provider organization should seek those from the potential country who have been educated in reservoir countries or (even better) who have been employed there or in transceiver countries as supervisors. These people can act as intercultural bridges. If such people are not available, personnel from the provider country will have to take top management responsibility, and set up more direct lines of reporting than they would at home.

2. Design
While potential country personnel will eventually assume design responsibility, this should not be expected *a priori*. All of the design work to adapt the process or product for technology transfer should be performed in the provider country. Frequently, a consultant from a reservoir country can speed the redesign. However, user-country personnel can grow into the design role by critiquing the proposed designs and making recommendations on which design aspects represent the greatest ease of assimilation, and which aspects should be changed to avoid assimilation problems.

3. Documentation
A still simpler level of documentation should be used than in Case A. Also, it may frequently be desirable to use physical techniques as alternates to documentation. These might include full-scale reference models, templates, or standardized reference cards. These can make it possible for useful work to be done by potential-nation personnel who cannot read or cannot interpret drawings. As mentioned previously, these manufacturing aids can be generated by a consultant.

Knobs, buttons and other controls should be labeled with symbols and/or the user's language. This should also be the case for operating instructions.

4. Manufacturing
In potential nations, manufacturing can rely far more heavily on labor-intensive techniques. This reduces dependence on complex equipment, increases employment, and may utilize manual skills which poten-

tial-country personnel possess at higher levels than those of personnel of reservoir or transceiver countries.

5. *Distribution/Service*
It is not reasonable to expect to create new networks for distribution and service in a potential country at the same time as introducing a new technology. The need to utilize what already exists must play a major role in the selection of the process or product to be transferred, even though improvements in distribution and service will take place over a longer period.

6. *End User*
The previous comments on end-user skills apply even more strongly, except for the possibility that the technology being transferred may be used to manufacture a product in the potential country, which will primarily be exported from it, to one where the end-users are already in tune with that product.

B. Materials

In addition to the need to use those materials available locally, environmental considerations are more critical than when a transceiver country is the user. Many of the potential countries have higher temperatures and humidity, and a relative scarcity of controlled atmospheres. These factors increase the rate of metal corrosion and the likelihood of fungal growth, and shorten the life of paints, coatings and adhesives. If environmental testing has not previously been done on all components of the product or process being transferred, such tests are a necessary first step in any technology transfer. Again, consultant testing services are valuable.

1. *Metals*
Since the variety of alloys will be more limited than when the user is a transceiver country, corrosion considerations are extremely important. A greater degree of over-design will be required, and particular attention must be paid to cleanliness, such as welding or brazing flux removal, elimination of water in confined spaces, etc., during metal fabrication.

2. *Chemicals*
The same comments apply as in Case A. Beyond that, not only will the choice of chemicals be more limited, but also it will be more difficult to obtain high-purity materials. If chemistry itself is the subject of technology transfer, consideration should be given to chemical plants using a large number of smaller modular elements, so that failure in any one area will not shut down the entire plant.

3. *Plastics and Composites*
One should expect to use forming processes with lower temperatures, pressures and precisions than in Case A. Epoxy-fiberglass is probably the only composite that should be considered.

4. Components

The level of components should be defined by locally available supplies. Fortunately, almost every country now has television, which means that those components necessary to repair television sets are likely to be available even in moderate-sized communities. Every effort should be made to design or redesign electronic products to take advantage of this level of components. In a similar way, mechanical products requiring standard components should take advantage of those used for readily available products such as bicycles, sewing machines, etc.

C. Methods

1. Fabrication

As remarked above, maximum use should be made of manual skills, simple tools and labor-intensive techniques. Over the longer term, increasing levels of equipment support, powered tools and automation may gradually be added, to the extent that they contribute improved productivity, improved quality or lower costs. In this way, they will also gradually improve the technological skills and knowledge base in the user country.

2. Assembly

Primary emphasis should be almost completely on mechanical assembly. However, productivity and accuracy can be increased with the use of simple assembly jigs and fixtures. Frequently these can be better defined by accepting suggestions from user-country personnel, rather than by using the preconceived ideas of representatives of the provider country. Periodic meetings for this purpose should be held as assembly familiarization takes place.

3. Testing

Simple go/no-go tests should be used wherever possible. Finished products should be put through operating tests, but it is also desirable to keep one or more "standard" products as references against which newly manufactured items can be compared.

IV. Case C: Reservoir to potential

Transfers from the most technical to the least technical nations have always seemed attractive. From the potential user's viewpoint, there is access to the most advanced capabilities. From the reservoir provider's viewpoint, there is a more open market. However, the wide gap means that the risks are greater than when transfers occur between countries that are technologically closer. For that reason, greater care and more thorough planning are required—and a consultant with experience in both provider and user countries can do much to assure success.

The risks arise because each participant may not know enough about the other. Reservoir management often expects a higher level of infrastructure than actually exists in the user country; potential users may not recognize the need for support requirements which the provider takes for granted.

There are many cases where transfers have failed. These range from initial acceptance but subsequent rejection of new agricultural practices, to "graveyards" of rusted construction equipment for which there were no spare parts, to expensive medical scanners that have sat in their shipping crates for years. These failures almost invariably result from lack of understanding (and lack of study) in the provider country with regard to what the user could assimilate. An important task for a consultant is to supply a "complete disclosure": that is, investigate all of the relevant factors on both sides of the transfer, and exhibit these to both participants.

When a potential nation desires technology for which the design skills reside in a reservoir nation, it may also be desirable for the reservoir nation to work with a transceiver country as an intermediary, supplying the latter with design and other technology information but allowing the transceiver personnel to adapt the management, manufacturing practices and design details to the ultimate user. As mentioned earlier, a reservoir-country consultant is also especially useful in transceiver-to-potential transfers.

A detailed listing of the skills, materials and methods need not be given here for Case C, as it will be a combination of the considerations in Cases A and B, with recognition that the gaps are greater than in either of those cases.

V. Practical matters

The necessary steps in a transfer will be determined by the chosen technology. However, outside of those steps, there are several practical matters that are often handled too lightly. We emphasize that they are as vital to success as the transfer itself.

A. Survey
In any transfer we strongly recommend that consultants and personnel from the provider country visit the user country for a long enough time to achieve an understanding of the available skills, materials and methods—as well as to recognize the infrastructure and attitudinal factors that are also so important in accepting any new technology.

B. Personnel Selection
The user-country personnel who are expected to play key roles in the technology transfer should be selected with great care. We recommend that candidate personnel visit the facilities in the provider country for several weeks, giving time for enough interchange between them and provider personnel to verify that they are capable of accepting the new

155

problems which technology transfer will bring. Consultants can set up procedures to review, test and screen these candidates.

C. Familiarization/Training
Designing, operating and manufacturing personnel from the user country should be in residence at the provider facility for several months at the initial stages of transfer, working in parallel with provider personnel. On their return to the user country, they should be accompanied by those provider personnel who will continue to work with them during the transfer and will also play a role in training other user personnel. These user personnel will become supervisors, and will form a cadre from which ideas and training can spread.

D. Communications and Review
We recommend every means possible to ensure frequent exchanges of ideas and information between provider and user personnel. Facsimile is superior to both telephone and teletypewriter, as it is freer from language difficulties and allows the direct exchange of written information in any script without the need for an operator's intervention. It also permits the transmission of sketches, drawing corrections, etc.

It is also vital for personnel to meet frequently. A schedule of visits alternating at each location should be set up in advance and strictly adhered to. These meetings provide an opportunity to review progress and problems and answer questions, solve personality problems, etc. It may be desirable to include a private third-party consultant or a representative of an international agency as a protective check on both sides and as an independent evaluator and arbitrator in case of disputes. Even after the transfer, we recommend that provider personnel visit the site periodically. Such visits can verify proper operation, answer newly arisen questions, and correct any unanticipated problems. Depending on the nature of the transfers, these can take place for up to four years.

VI. Facilitators

By facilitators, we mean agencies separate either from the provider or from the user. One type of facilitator is financial. Personnel from the funding agency can help to set up estimates of costs and rates of expenditure against which subsequent progress can be judged. They can also seek additional funds in the event of difficulties.

Educational institutions, especially within the user country, are important facilitators. Not only can they supply technical knowledge before and during the transfer, but also they can teach the skills needed by future staff. They should be contacted at the earliest stages.

International agencies are another type of facilitator. They can provide a valuable advisory rôle, frequently calling on a wide spectrum of experience and expertise. They can act to reassure skeptics in both the provider and the user countries, and in the financial community. We recommend that, even when arrangements have been made directly between the two parties to a technology transfer, an advisory link be set up with an international agency.

Finally, consultants can be valuable as facilitators. In addition to the technology and skills which they contribute, they can do much to communicate, to settle disputes, and to provide continual overall evaluation of a project. But they can do these things only if all parties accept that the consultants are fair in their judgements and truly dedicated to successful project completion.

In this paper, we have emphasized many problem areas, with the purpose of making sure that they can be solved. We are firmly convinced that, if the problems are properly addressed, technology transfer can be accomplished successfully, to the user nation's immense benefit.

CLOSING OF THE CONFERENCE

F. Vilardell
President, CIOMS

Mr Chairman, it is a great pleasure to bring this XXIIIrd CIOMS Conference to a close. From the excellent contributions and the discussions that have followed during these two days of hard work, it is obvious that health technology transfer is an extremely important and timely subject, for the nations that are receiving it as well as for the more fortunate, which are able to generate and distribute the most sophisticated instruments and procedures.

I am a citizen of Spain, a country that is somewhere in the middle, receiving technology, on the one hand, and donating some, on the other. Many of the problems that have been discussed here are familiar to me since they also present themselves at home. I hope that this conference will result in the establishment of some kind of more permanent body to further discuss the issues and help us in making decisions in our very different settings and perspectives.

May I congratulate the Chairman, Professor Ada, for conducting these sessions with such efficiency, including occasional firmness. The results of the arduous preparatory work by the programme committee are evident. The role of CIOMS as a catalyst for conferences like this makes it possible to assemble the best people to discuss each specialized subject. This has been certainly the case on this occasion.

We must thank the Director-General of WHO, Dr Nakajima, and the Deputy Director-General, Dr Abdelmoumène not only for facilitating the intellectual collaboration of WHO but also for its economic support, which has been essential for the success of the meeting. We thank also the officers of WHO who have collaborated closely in the preparation of this Conference: Drs Hanson, Mansourian and Szczerban.

May I thank again Dr Bankowski and the members of the CIOMS secretariat, Mrs Kathryn Chalaby-Amsler and Mrs Christine Düberdorfer, for their invaluable help.

The XXIIIrd CIOMS Conference is now adjourned.

LIST OF PARTICIPANTS

ABDELMOUMENE, M. Deputy Director-General, WHO, Geneva

ABDUSSALAM, M. Bundesgesundheitsamt, Berlin, Federal Republic of Germany

ABONDO, A. Institute of Medical Research and Studies of Medicinal Plants, Yaoundé, Republic of Cameroon

ADA, G.L. The John Curtin School of Medical Research, Canberra, Australia

ADEKUNLE, O. Confederation of African Medical Associations and Societies, Ibadan, Nigeria

AKERELE, C.O. Traditional Medicine, WHO, Geneva

AL-RIFAI, A. Kuwait Institute for Medical Specializations, Kuwait

AL-SAIF, A. Islamic Organization for Medical Sciences, Kuwait

ARNOLD, R.B. International Federation of Pharmaceutical Manufacturers Associations, Geneva, Switzerland

ASSI-ADOU, J. Paediatric Department, Faculty of Medicine, Abidjan, Côte d'Ivoire

ATTINGER, E.O. School of Engineering and Applied Science and School of Medicine, University of Virginia, Charlottesville, VA, U.S.A.

BADRAN, I.G. The Egyptian Academy of Scientific Research and Technology, Cairo, Egypt

BAKER, B. International Union Against Cancer, Geneva, Switzerland

BANKOWSKI, Z. Council for International Organizations of Medical Sciences, Geneva

BATU, Aung Than. WHO Regional Office for South-East Asia, New Delhi, India

BECHER, E. Organisation for Economic Cooperation and Development, Paris, France

BEKTIMIROV, T. Assistant Director-General, WHO, Geneva

BELCHIOR, M. Council for International Organizations of Medical Sciences, Geneva

BERDJIS, C.C. International Council of Societies of Pathology, Geneva, Switzerland

BIANCO, N. Centro Nacional de Immunoligia Clinica, Venezuela

BINGOL, G. Ministry of Health, Sihhiye/Ankara, Turkey

BIRCHER, J. International Association for the Study of the Liver, Göttingen, Federal Republic of Germany

BLAND, J.H. Programme Support Service, WHO, Geneva

BOGEL, K. Veterinary Public Health, WHO, Geneva

BOSEILA, A.-W. The Egyptian Academy of Scientific Research and Technology, Cairo, Egypt

BRAEHMER, H. Standing Representation of the German Democratic Republic at the Office of the United Nations and Other International Organizations in Geneva, Geneva, Switzerland

BRAVEN, R. International Confederation of Midwives, Lausanne, Switzerland de BRUYCKER, M. Tropical Medicine Subprogramme of "Science and Technology for Development", Commission of the European Communities, Brussels, Belgium

BRYANT, J. H. Department of Community Health Sciences, Aga Khan University, Karachi, Pakistan

BUCH ANDREASEN, P. Danish Medical Research Council; International Society of Technology Assessment in Health Care, Hellerup, Denmark

BULYZHENKOV, V. Hereditary Diseases Programme, WHO, Geneva

CAMERON, C. Forensic and Research Services, Department of National Health and Population Development, Pretoria, Republic of South Africa

CAPRON, A. M. The Law Center, University of Southern California, Los Angeles, California, U.S.A.

CASTILLO, G. University of the Philippines at Los Banos, Philippines

CHIGAN, E. Noncommunicable Diseases and Health Technology, WHO, Geneva

CHRZANOWSKI, R. Swiss Institute of Public Health and Hospitals, Federal Office of Public Health, Aarau, Switzerland

CLEMENT, P. International Rhinologic Society, Brussels, Belgium

COURVOISIER, B. Académie suisse des Sciences médicales, Geneva, Switzerland

DANIELSSON, H. The Swedish Medical Research Council, Stockholm, Sweden

DAVIES, A. M. School of Public Health, Hebrew University, Jerusalem, Israel

DEOM, A. International Federation of Clinical Chemistry, Geneva, Switzerland

DICHTER, D. Technology for the People, Geneva, Switzerland

DIENG, B. Institut de Recherche de Biologie Appliquée, Kindia, République de Guinée

DION, P. World Veterans Federation, Surrey, United Kingdom

EDEN, M. Biomedical Engineering and Instrumentation Branch, National Institutes of Health, Bethesda, Maryland, U.S.A.

ELIS, J. Czechoslovak Academy of Sciences, Prague, Czecholovakia

ESPERANCA PINA, J. Scientific Council for Health Sciences, Instituto Nacional de Investigacao Cientifica, Lisbon, Portugal

FATTORUSSO, V. Drug Management and Policies, WHO, Geneva

FIORI, L. Comité international catholique des Infirmières et Assistantes Medico Sociales, Vatican City, Italy

FUTTERKNECHT, A. Industry Council for Development (New York), Möhlin, Switzerland

GALLAGHER, J. Council for International Organizations of Medical Sciences, Geneva

de GEER, G. International Society of Radiology, Geneva, Switzerland

GEZAIRY, H. A. WHO Regional Office for the Eastern Mediterranean, Alexandria, Egypt

GIBBS, W. Health Laboratory Technology and Blood Safety, WHO, Geneva

GODAL, T. Special Programme for Research and Training in Tropical Diseases, WHO, Geneva

GOON, E. Development of Human Resources for Health, WHO, Geneva

GOPALAN, C. Nutrition Foundation of India, New Delhi

GORNICKI, B. Federation of Medical Societies of Poland, Warsaw, Poland

GUIDOTTI, R. Maternal and Child Health, WHO, Geneva

GYARFAS, I. Cardiovascular Diseases, WHO, Geneva

HACHEN, H.J. International Rehabilitation Medicine Association, Geneva, Switzerland

HAG-ALI, M. Medical Research Council, Khartoum, Sudan

HALL, P. Special Programme of Research, Development and Research Training in Human Reproduction, WHO, Geneva

HANSON, G. Radiation Medicine, WHO, Geneva

HAPSARA, H. Division of Epidemiological Surveillance and Health Situation and Trend Assessment, WHO, Geneva

HASSAR, M. Institut National d'Hygiène, Rabat, Morocco

HEUCK, C. Health Laboratory Technology and Blood Safety, WHO, Geneva

HOET, J.J. International Diabetes Federation, Brussels, Belgium

HU, Ching-Li. Assistant Director-General, WHO, Geneva

HU, D.J. Expanded Programme on Immunization, WHO, Geneva

HUCH, A. Universitätsspital Zürich, Frauenklinik, Dept. Geburtshilfe, Zürich, Switzerland

INOUYE, E. Science Council of Japan, Tokyo, Japan

ISSAKOV, A. National Health Systems and Policies, WHO, Geneva

JØRGENSEN, Torben. International Federation for Medical and Biological Engineering, Danish Hospital Institute, Copenhagen, Denmark

JARDEL, J.-P. Assistant Director-General, WHO, Geneva

JOHANNISSON, E. International Federation of Fertility Societies, Geneva, Switzerland

JOHNSEN, D. U.S. Permanent Mission to the United Nations Office at Geneva, Geneva, Switzerland

KABANO, A. Ministry of Health, Kigali, Rwanda

KAIHARA, S. Hospital Computer Center, University of Tokyo Hospital, Tokyo, Japan

KALLINGS, L.O. Ministry of Health and Social Affairs, Stockholm, Sweden

KASEJE, D. Christian Medical Commission, World Council of Churches, Geneva, Switzerland

KAWAGUCHI, Y. Planning, Coordination and Cooperation, WHO, Geneva

KERN, A. Division of Public Information, WHO, Geneva

KHAN, Amanullah, Pakistan Medical Research Council, Lahore, Pakistan

KHAN, I. Psychotropic and Narcotic Drugs, WHO, Geneva

KHONJE, P.R. Ministry of Health, Lilongwe, Malawi

KLIOUKINE, I. Inter-Parliamentary Union, Geneva, Switzerland

KOCH, P. Swiss Federal Office of Social Insurances, Bern, Switzerland

KOCHI, A. Tuberculosis, WHO, Geneva

KOLENOGLU, S.Z. Ministry of Health, Ankara, Turkey

KORTE, R. German Agency for Technical Cooperation (GTZ), Escborn, Federal Republic of Germany

KOSTRZEWSKI, J. Polish Academy of Sciences, Warsaw, Poland

LAROCHE, C. Fédération internationale du Thermalisme et du Climatisme, Paris, France

LAZARO, P. Ministerio de Sanidad y Consumo, Madrid, Spain

LEENEN, H.J.J. Royal Dutch Academy of Sciences, Amsterdam, The Netherlands

LEMMÉ, H. Federal Health Office, Berlin, Federal Republic of Germany

LETOURNEAU, E. Bureau of Radiation and Medical Devices, Health and Welfare Canada, Ottawa, Ontario, Canada

LIISBERG, E. World Health Forum, WHO, Geneva

LOMMEL, H. World Association of Societies of Pathology (Anatomic and Clinical), Leverkusen, Federal Republic of Germany

LOPEZ, C. Health Laboratory Technology and Blood Safety, WHO, Geneva

MAGRATH, D. Biologicals, WHO, Geneva

MAGYAR, K. Federation of Hungarian Medical Societies, Budapest, Hungary

MAKELA, P.H. Academy of Finland, National Public Health Institute, Helsinki, Finland

MALCOLM, L. Community Health Department, University of Otago, Wellington, New Zealand

MALLOUPPAS, A. WHO Collaborating Centre for Training and Research on Maintenance and Repair of Health Care Equipment/Higher Technical Institute, Nicosia, Cyprus

MANDIL, S. Information Systems Support, WHO, Geneva

MANSOURIAN, B. Research Promotion and Development, WHO, Geneva

MARQUET, J.F. International Federation of Otorhinolaryngological Societies, Berchem, Belgium

MARUOTTI, R. International College of Surgeons, Milan, Italy

MESDAGHINIA, A. School of Public Health, Tehran University of Medical Sciences, Tehran, Iran

METTERS, J. Department of Health, London, England

MICHELSEN, J. Instituto Nacional de Salud, Bogota, Colombia

MIYAMOTO, M. Ministry of Health, Brasilia, Brazil

MOATTI, J.-P. "Evaluation des risques et des Actions de Prévention", INSERM, Paris, France

MONTALBETTI, N. International Union of Pure and Applied Chemistry, Milan, Italy

MONTELL, R. Finnida, Helsinki, Finland

MOORE, J.F. Bio-Imaging Research, Inc., Lincolnshire, Illinois, U.S.A.

MOTZEL, C. Medical Women's International Association, Cologne, Federal Republic of Germany

NAJERA-MORRONDO, J.A. Malaria Action Programme, WHO, Geneva

NAKAJIMA, H. Director-General, WHO, Geneva

NATHANSON, V. Commonwealth Medical Association, London, England

NOBEL, J. ECRI, Plymouth Meeting, Pennsylvania, U.S.A.

NORTON, C. Global Programme on AIDS, WHO, Geneva

O'GORMAN, V. Health Research Board, Dublin, Ireland

O'HARE, M. World Confederation for Physical Therapy, London, England

OGUISSA, T. International Council of Nurses, Geneva, Switzerland

OLIECH, J.S. Medical Services, Ministry of Health, Nairobi, Kenya

OSUNTOKUN, B.O. School of Medicine, University of Ibadan, Ibadan, Nigeria

PALMER, P.E.S. Department of Radiology, University of California, Davis, California, U.S.A.

PENA, Jorge. Pan American Health Organization, WHO Regional Office for the Americas, Washington, D.C., U.S.A.

POORWO SOEDARMO, S. National Institute of Health Research and Development, Ministry of Health, Jakarta, Republic of Indonesia

PRADILLA, A. Nutrition, WHO, Geneva

QUAMINA, E.S.M. External Impact Evaluation of Special Programme of Research, Development and Research Training in Human Reproduction; Population Council, Trinidad & Tobago, West Indies

de RAADT, P. Parasitic Diseases Programme, WHO, Geneva

RACOVEANU, N.T. WHO Regional Office for Europe, Copenhagen, Denmark

RAY, D. Office of Governing Bodies and Protocol, WHO, Geneva

REESE, K. World Federation of Proprietary Medicine Manufacturers, Bonn, Federal Republic of Germany

RESTREPO, M. Instituto Nacional de Salud, Bogota, Colombia

REY, P. International Ergonomics Association, Geneva, Switzerland

RICHARD, C. United Nations, Geneva, Switzerland

RIFKA, G.E., Eastern Mediterranean Special Programme, WHO, Geneva

RO, Kong-Kyun. Department of Management Science, Korea Advanced Institute of Science and Technology, Seoul, Korea

ROCHE, L. World Federation of Associations of Clinical Toxicology Centers and Poison Control Centers, Lyon, France

RODRIGUEZ-FARRE, E. Consejo Superior de Investigaciones Cientificas, Madrid, Spain

ROZEE, K. Bureau of Microbiology, Laboratory Centre for Disease Control, Health & Welfare Canada, Ottawa, Ontario, Canada

RUSSBACH, R. International Committee of the Red Cross, Geneva, Switzerland

RUTISHAUSER, W. International Society and Federation of Cardiology, Geneva, Switzerland

SANKARAN, B. St. Stephens Hospital, New Delhi, India

SARGENTINI, A. Laboratory of Biomedical Engineering, Instituto Superiore di Sanità, Rome, Italy

SARTORIUS, N. Division of Mental Health, WHO, Geneva

SAWADOGO, M. Institut de Recherche sur les Substances Naturelles, Ouagadougou, Burkina Faso

SAYERS, B. McA. Centre for Cognitive Systems, Imperial College, London, England

SCHIØLER, G. National Board of Health, Copenhagen, Denmark

SCHROEDER, M. Collège médical, Bridel, Grand-Duchy of Luxemburg

de SCOVILLE, A. Comité des Académies royales de Médecine de Belgique, Brussels, Belgium

SEHR, A. Association of the Czechoslovak Medical Societies J. E. Purkyne, Prague, Czechoslovakia

SENN, A. International College of Angiology, Bern, Switzerland

SICKMULLER, B. Bundesverband der Pharmazutishen Industrie (BPI), Frankfurt, Federal Republic of Germany

SIIM, J. C. The Royal Danish Academy of Sciences and Letters, Copenhagen, Denmark

SOEDARMO, S. P. National Institute of Health Research and Development, Jakarta, Indonesia

SOLBAKK, J. H. Council for Medical Research, The Norwegian Research Council for Science and Humanities, Oslo, Norway

STJERNSWARD, J. Cancer and Palliative Care, WHO, Geneva

STRASSER, T. World Hypertension League, Geneva, Switzerland

SURYANARAYNA, L. Andhra Pradesh University of Health Sciences, Andhra Pradesh, India

SZCZERBAN, J. Research Promotion and Development, WHO, Geneva

THANGARAJ, R. H. Council for International Organizations of Medical Sciences, Salur, India

TONGUE, A. International Council on Alcohol and Addictions, Lausanne, Switzerland

TORRIGIANI, G. Division of Communicable Diseases, WHO, Geneva

TRENS, FLORES, E. Unidad de Desarrollo Tecnologico, Facultad de Medicina, Mexico, D. F., Mexico

VALENTIN, J.-M. International Union of Architects, Public Health Group, Neuilly, France

VAN PERNIS, A. World Federation of Public Health Associations, Geneva, Switzerland

VENULET, J. Council for International Organizations of Medical Sciences, Geneva

VERWILGHEN, R. L. International Committee for Standardization of Haematology, Leuven, Belgium

VIGNES, C. H. Office of the Legal Counsel, WHO, Geneva

VILARDELL, F. Council for International Organization of Medical Sciences, Barcelona, Spain

VILLFORTH, J. C. Center for Devices and Radiological Health, Food and Drug Administration, Bethesda, Maryland, U.S.A.

VIOLAKI-PARASKEVA, M. Ethics and Medical Association of Greece, Athens, Greece

VIVES-CORRONS, J. L. International Society of Haematology (European and African Division), Barcelona, Spain

VOLODIN, V. Radiation Medicine, WHO, Geneva

WACKENHEIM, A. Collège d'Enseignement Post-Universitaire de Radiologie, Strasbourg, France

WALDVOGEL, F. University Hospital, Clinique médicale thérapeutique, Geneva, Switzerland

WASUNNA, A. Clinical Technology, WHO, Geneva

WAUGH, M. International Union against the Venereal Diseases and the Treponematoses, Leeds, England

WIDDUS, R. Global Programme on AIDS, WHO, Geneva

WOOD, C. African Medical & Research Foundation, Nairobi, Kenya

WYNEN, A. World Medical Association, Braine l'Alleud, Belgium

YAKIN, G. Ministry of Health, Ankara, Turkey

ZAIMOV, K. Union of the Scientific Medical Societies, Sofia, Bulgaria

ZARKOVIC, G. Committee on Health Care, Academy of Sciences and Arts, Sarajevo, Yugoslavia